A STEP-BY-STEP GUIDE TO

SHIATSU

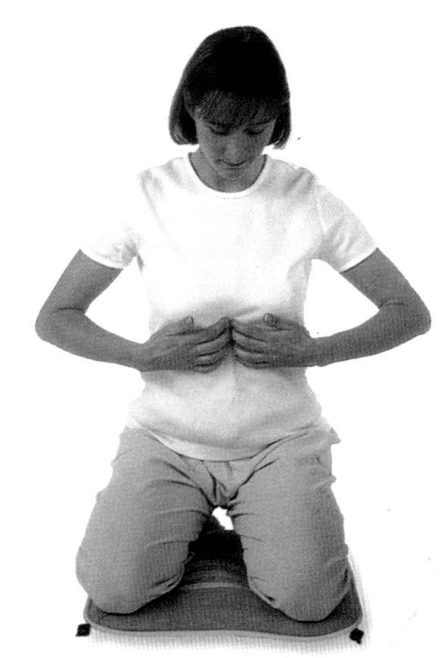

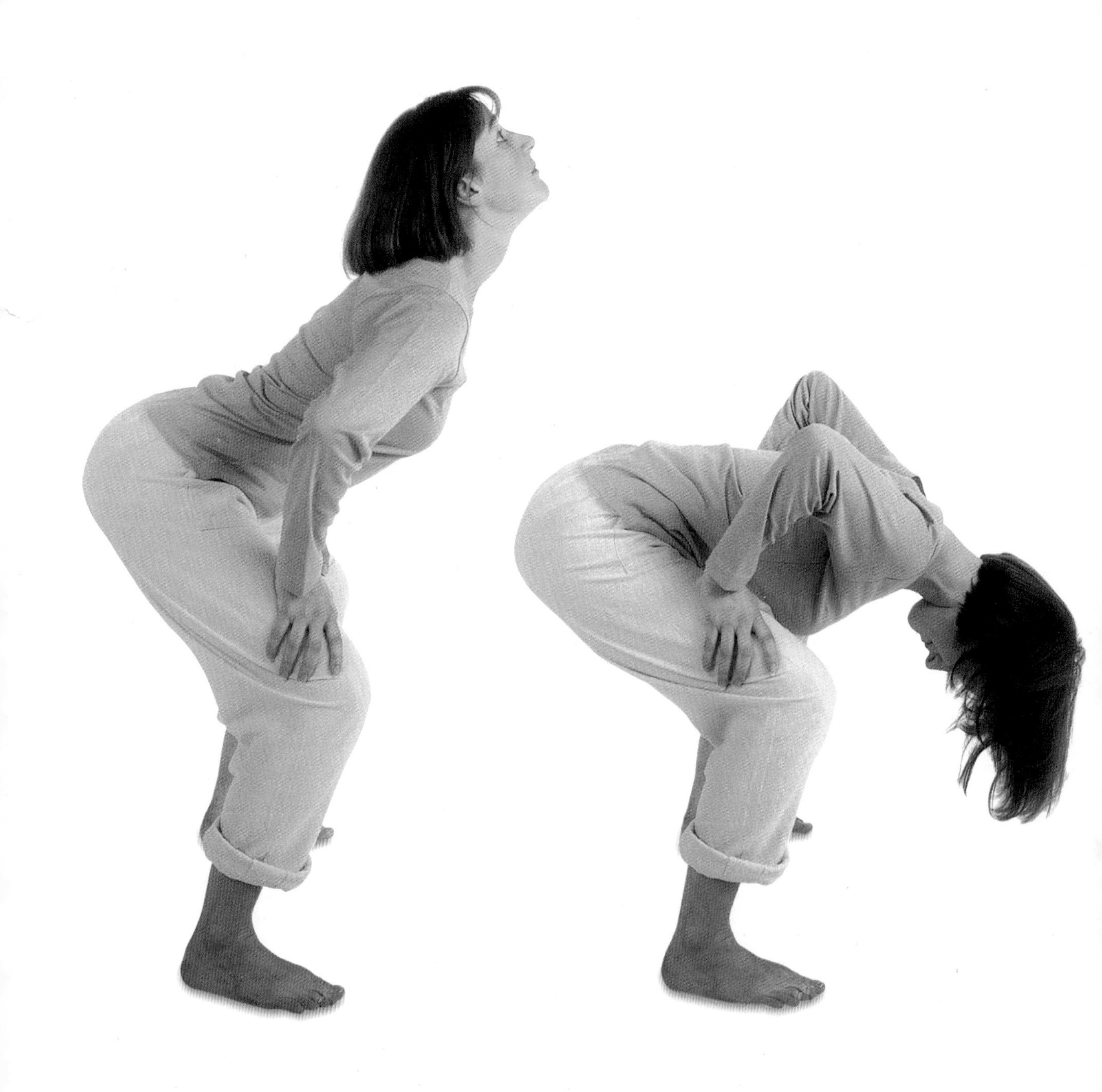

A STEP-BY-STEP GUIDE TO

SHIATSU

a simple introduction to the ancient therapy of pressure and nurturing touch, with 170 easy-to-follow photographs

Susanne Franzen

Special Photography Don Last

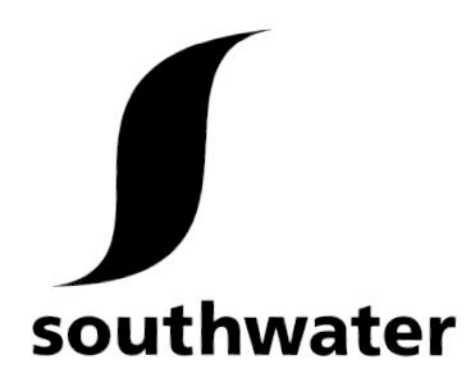

This edition is published by Southwater, an imprint of Anness Publishing Ltd,
Hermes House, 88–89 Blackfriars Road, London SE1 8HA;
tel. 020 7401 2077; fax 020 7633 9499
www.southwaterbooks.com; www.annesspublishing.com

If you like the images in this book and would like to investigate
using them for publishing, promotions or advertising, please
visit our website www.practicalpictures.com for more information.

UK agent: The Manning Partnership Ltd;
tel. 01225 478444; fax 01225 478440; sales@manning-partnership.co.uk
UK distributor: Grantham Book Services Ltd;
tel. 01476 541080; fax 01476 541061; orders@gbs.tbs-ltd.co.uk
North American agent/distributor: National Book Network;
tel. 301 459 3366; fax 301 429 5746; www.nbnbooks.com
Australian agent/distributor: Pan Macmillan Australia;
tel. 1300 135 113; fax 1300 135 103; customer.service@macmillan.com.au
New Zealand agent/distributor: David Bateman Ltd;
tel. (09) 415 7664; fax (09) 415 8892

Publisher: Joanna Lorenz
Project Editor: Fiona Eaton
Designer: Allan Mole
Photographer: Don Last

ETHICAL TRADING POLICY

Because of our ongoing ecological investment programme, you, as our customer, can have the pleasure and reassurance of knowing that a tree is being cultivated on your behalf to naturally replace the materials used to make the book you are holding. For further information about this scheme, go to www.annesspublishing.com/trees

A CIP catalogue record for this book is available from the British Library.

Previously published as *Shiatsu for Health and Well-Being*

PUBLISHER'S NOTE

The reader should not regard the recommendations, ideas and techniques expressed and described in this book as substitutes for the advice of a qualified medical practitioner or other qualified professional. Any use to which the recommendations, ideas and techniques are put is at the reader's sole discretion and risk.

CONTENTS

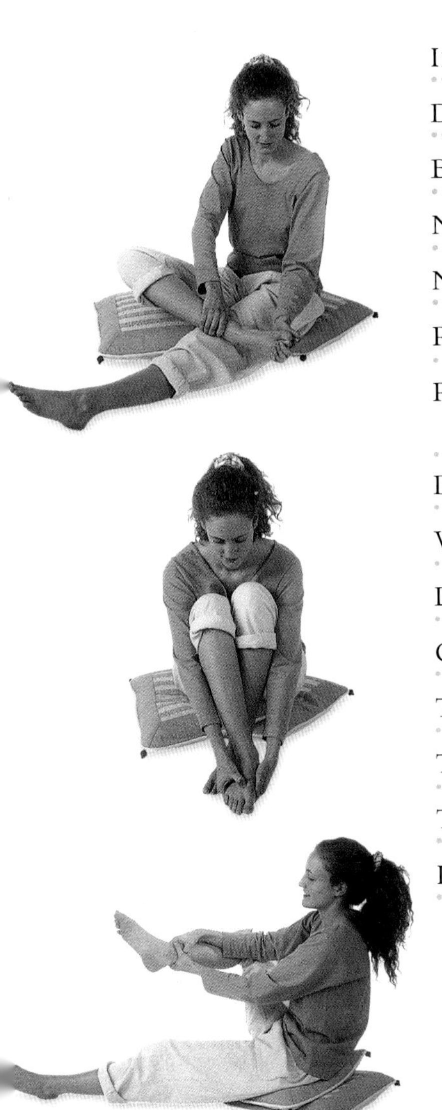

WHAT IS SHIATSU?

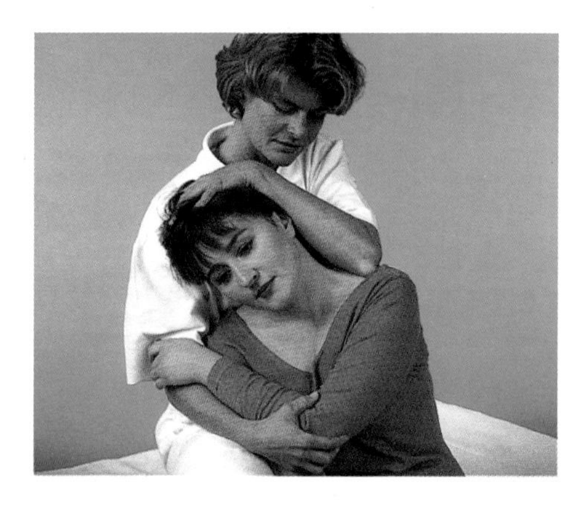

Touch is the essence of Shiatsu. We all need to be touched in some form, and Shiatsu gives you a wonderful opportunity to fulfil this need in a loving and caring way. The nurturing touch of Shiatsu helps trigger the self-healing process within.

Shiatsu is a physical therapy aimed at treating your condition through the application of touch as well as helping you to learn how to heal yourself. The treatment approach and philosophy is similar to acupuncture in its usage of the meridians (energy channels) and *tsubo* (pressure points) but Shiatsu does not call for needles.

"Shiatsu" is a Japanese word meaning "finger pressure". The application of pressure is the underlying principle of Shiatsu. Different stretching techniques and corrective exercises may also be part of the treatment with the intention of creating balance in the body, both physically and energetically.

It is easy to learn the basic principles of Shiatsu; it is also enjoyable and makes you feel good. You are taking responsibility for your own health, and taking care of yourself is very important, as it empowers you to create changes when needed. Combine the DoIn exercises illustrated in this book with the different self-treatment techniques to improve your physical and mental health and well-being. Take some "time out" and give your partner or a friend a Shiatsu treatment, allowing both of you space for reflection and rest. You will feel the benefits of Shiatsu both as a giver and a receiver.

In Shiatsu we take a holistic approach and look at the whole person – body, mind and spirit – in trying to find out where the imbalances and causes for the stress lie.

- In Shiatsu we use the power of touch to relieve aches and pains and to help relax both the body and the mind.
- Shiatsu creates a greater self-awareness and gives an understanding of how your body reacts to stress and what you can do to prevent this happening.
- Shiatsu will strengthen the body's own self-defence and by doing so, improve your general health and well-being, physically and emotionally.

A State of Balance

Yin and Yang

Balance, or the lack thereof, is an important focus in the Shiatsu approach to health. The single most fundamental principle of Shiatsu and Eastern medicine is the concept of Yin and Yang. Yin and Yang represent two opposite yet complementary aspects in nature. Everything is essentially composed of and affected by these two forces and naturally grouped into complementary pairs of opposites. The table shows some examples of Yin and Yang qualities.

Yin	*Yang*
Earth	Heaven
Darkness	Light
Passive	Active
Open	Closed
Soft	Hard
Female	Male
Front	Back
Interior	Exterior
Cold	Hot
Water	Fire

Because Yin and Yang are complementary forces, nothing in nature is solely Yin or Yang; everything and everyone is composed of both in varying degrees. In a dark night (Yin) there will be bright stars (Yang) in the sky. At the same time nothing is neutral; either Yin or Yang predominates. The key to health is to try to create a balance between the forces; to be able to activate our muscles and brain during the lighter part of the day (Yang qualities) and then allow for relaxation, stillness and rest when the darkness sets in (Yin qualities).

Yin and Yang tells us about a process of change. Everything changes all the time; nothing is completely still. Day turns to night and back to day again. Everything has a cycle and Yin and Yang merely show how energy is moving in one way or the other.

Ki – Energy

Shiatsu works on this flow of energy or "Ki", that circulates through our bodies in specific pathways called meridians. Ki is a fundamental concept in Eastern medical thinking and we consider it as our "life essence", which maintains and nurtures our physical body and therefore also affects our mind and spirit. The "life force" is responsible for the creation of our physical body and maintains an inner homeostatic balance in the body. The flow of Ki through the meridians can be disturbed in different ways: either by external traumas, such as an injury, or internal traumas such as anxiety or stress. This is when aches and pains and similar symptoms start to occur and you may experience discomfort mentally and/or physically. In Shiatsu we use touch to assess the disturbed flow of Ki in the body and try to correct any imbalances accordingly.

THE MERIDIANS

ORGANS - MERIDIANS

The balanced functioning of our body is controlled by twelve vital internal Organs. In Oriental medicine the Organs have a wider meaning than in the West, based on their physiological and energetic function. The Organs do not simply consist of their physical structures; each has a different quality of energetic movement and responsibility. The functions of the twelve vital Organs are listed here. The use of capital letters differentiates the Oriental interpretation of an Organ from its Western equivalent.

Each of the twelve Organs is linked to a meridian, or energy channel, named according to the internal Organ it affects. The meridians run in pairs either side of the body, they ensure nurturing of Ki.

TSUBO – PRESSURE POINTS

Along each meridian are a varying number of *tsubo,* or pressure points. They are points along the meridian where the energy is thought to be flowing near the surface of the body and therefore more accessible for treatment. There are more than 700 *tsubo* in your body and they are numbered in sequence according to which meridian they are on. The first point on the Kidney meridian, for example, will be Kidney 1 (KID 1). The points reflect the internal functioning of the body and can be used for both diagnosis and treatment purposes.

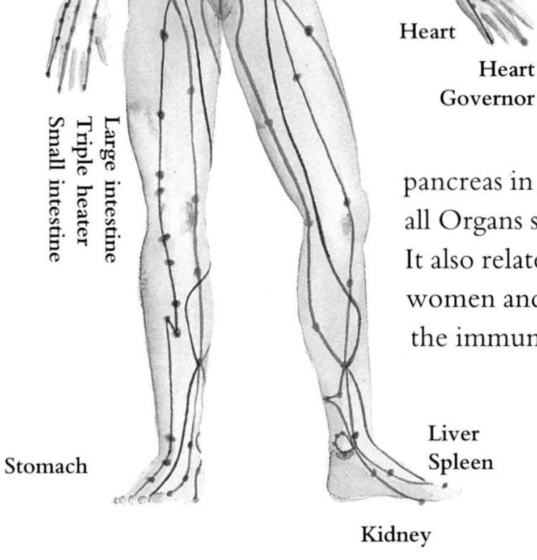

Lungs (LU):

- Take in air and vital Ki during respiration to refine and distribute it around the body. A fundamental process for building up resistance against external intrusions.
- Elimination of gases through exhalation.
- Openness, emotional stability, enthusiasm and positivity.

Large Intestine (LI):

- Helps the function of the Lungs. Processes food substances and eliminates what is unnecessary.
- The ability to "let go". Elimination.

Spleen (SP):

- Corresponds to the function of the pancreas in Western terms and governs all Organs secreting digestive enzymes. It also relates to reproductive glands in women and is a controlling factor in the immune system.
- Maintains the health of the flesh, the connective soft tissue and the muscle tissue.

• Self-image is strongly affected by the Spleen function and the desire to help others is apparent. Self-confident.

Stomach (ST):

• Responsible for "receiving and ripening" ingested food and fluids.

• Information for mental and physical nourishment.

• Well-grounded, centred, self-confident and reliable.

Heart (HT):

• Governs blood and blood vessels; circulatory system.

• Houses the Mind and our emotions.

• Joyful, calm and communicative.

Small Intestine (SI):

• The quality of the blood and tissue reflects the condition of the Small Intestine, and anxiety, emotional excitement or nervous shock can adversely affect the Small Intestine energy.

• Emotional stability and calmness.

Kidneys (KID):

• The Kidneys include the function of the adrenals, controlling the whole of the hormonal system.

• Provides and stores essential Ki for all other organs and governs birth, growth, reproduction and development; the reproductive system.

• Nourishes the spine, bones and the brain; the nervous system.

• Vitality, direction, courage and will power.

Bladder (BL):

• Purification and regulation.

• Nourishes the spine.

• Gives courage and ability to move forward in life.

Heart Governor (HG):

• Protector of the heart and closely related to emotional responses.

• Related to central circulation.

• Influences relationships with others; protective of others.

Triple Heater (TH):

• Transports energy, blood and heat to the peripheral parts of the body; circulatory system.

• Helpful and emotionally interactive.

Liver (LIV):

• Stores blood and nutrients which are subsequently distributed throughout the body. Ensures free flow of Ki throughout the body.

• Governs the muscular and digestive systems.

• Creative and full of ideas; good planning and organization.

Gall Bladder (GB):

• Stores bile produced by the Liver and distributes it in the Small Intestine; digestive system.

• Practical application of ideas and decision-making.

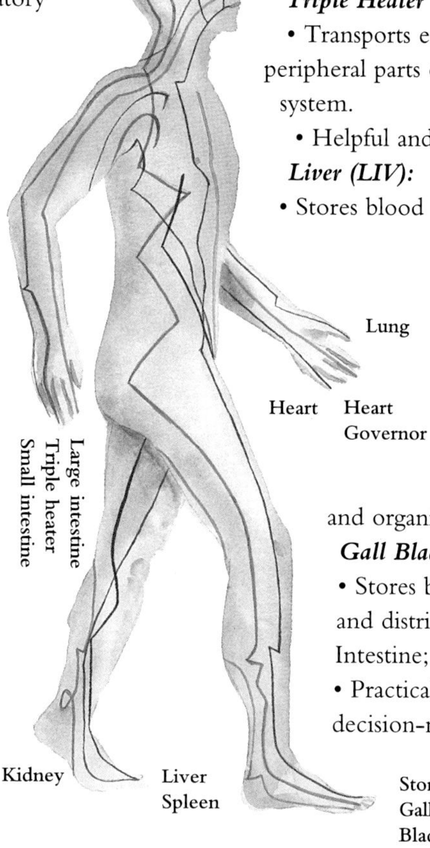

Stress: A Cause of Imbalance

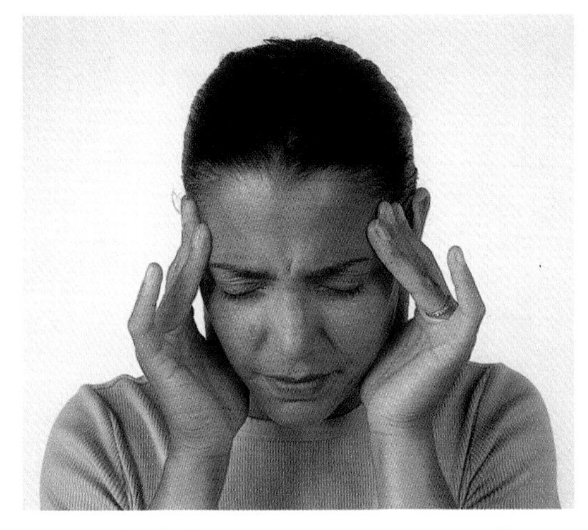
Tension headaches are a common symptom of stress.

Stress upsets both your mental and physical well-being, and every one of us has felt its grasp at one time or another. Stress is well known to all Shiatsu practitioners and is recognized as one of the major factors affecting health in our modern society. It is a normal part of life; in fact a certain amount of stress is good for us. Some people seem to be able to thrive on it, yet for others the pressure can be too much. The cumulative impact of events sometimes means that, eventually, we cannot cope. The pressure becomes overpowering and we begin to react to the stress in different ways. These reactions will affect our health and well-being and may interfere with our jobs and our social lives in a negative way. The body reacts to a stressor with first a diminished, then an increased, level of resistance. This is usually called the "fight or flight" reaction, which gives responses in all the systems in our body.

Stress, with all its different symptoms, is a sign that we have lost balance in our life. Human beings have a wonderful natural system for maintaining balance, and the body is always striving to achieve this state of balance and inner harmony. It is this balancing adaptive energy that is tested by stress, and which is constantly under challenge. Coping with stress can be made easier by asking for help and support from family and friends. Talking to someone helps you to see a problem more clearly.

Far better than just talking, however, having someone give you a Shiatsu treatment will relax your body and mind and bring back a sense of general well-being.

Fight or Flight Response

- The brain registers danger and sends messages along the nerves to different muscles and organs to react accordingly (nervous/muscular system).
- The heart beats faster, pumping out blood to muscles and areas in need and you start to sweat (circulatory system).
- The breathing rhythm changes; you start to breathe faster due to more air being drawn in through the bronchial tubes as they expand (respiratory system).
- The digestion slows down (digestive system).
- Increased production of certain hormones, such as adrenalin and noradrenalin (hormonal system).

A Balanced Lifestyle

You can improve general health and well-being and your defences by understanding what causes you stress and by learning how to avoid it or adapt to it. There are basically two aspects to stress reduction: lifestyle modification and relaxation.

Lifestyle modification could mean changing your job and reassessing your goals in life or simply adapting a more open attitude to what you are doing. Having a sense of control over events lessens their stressful impact.

Daily relaxation represents the most important element of maintaining health and vitality. Deep relaxation is not the same as sleep, and to gain full benefit from it, it is important not to fall asleep while relaxing. Giving or receiving a Shiatsu treatment will relax your whole body and mind and you will feel totally refreshed and energized afterwards.

Try to eat a well-balanced diet rich in fibres, grains and fresh vegetables; cut down on sugar and salt as well as coffee, tea and carbonated soft drinks.

A certain amount of physical exercise is necessary if you want to maintain your health and vitality. A pleasant, brisk 20-minute walk in the fresh air every day will stimulate and balance the energy within, or try to include the DoIn session at least once in your daily routine. The important thing is that the exercise you choose should feel pleasurable – which for some of us can be a problem.

Left: Exercise will enhance your vitality.

Below: A well-balanced diet, rich in fruit and vegetables, is essential for health.

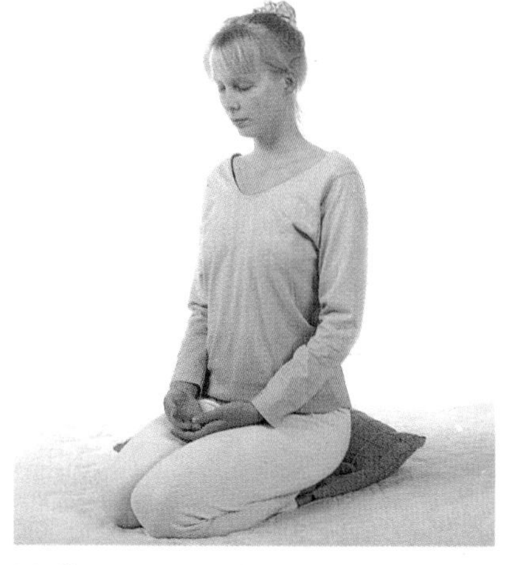

Meditation is a good relaxation technique.

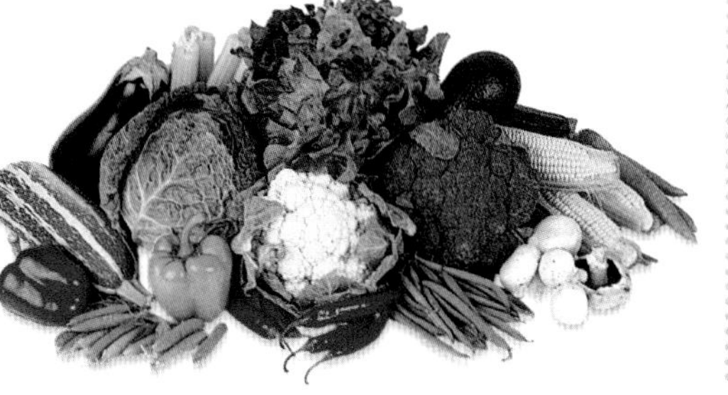

Shiatsu with a Partner

Giving and receiving Shiatsu is both enjoyable and relaxing and a wonderful way of spending time with another person. An important consideration in giving Shiatsu is how to touch. Different people, different signs and symptoms, require a different quality of touch and treatment approach. Your touch needs to be very light for some energy "listening" techniques and very firm for deep tissue work. Try to use your hands as an extension of your heart, and be sensitive to your partner's needs.

You can give and receive Shiatsu as frequently as you wish. There are times, however, when Shiatsu is not appropriate or when someone should be referred to a professional therapist for expert advice and treatment. In any case, *use your common sense.*

Before you Begin

You need to consider your health and condition before giving a Shiatsu treatment. You should not give Shiatsu if you are tired or intoxicated, have a contagious disease or if for any reason you do not feel up to it. Before you start, it is important to think about the environment. The space should be clean, warm and comforting without any noise in the background.

Caution

Do not give Shiatsu if your partner:

- has a high fever
- is intoxicated
- is suffering from chronic blood pressure - refer to a doctor
- has blood-borne cancer
- is in the first three months of pregnancy - refer to a professional Shiatsu practitioner
- has a contagious disease

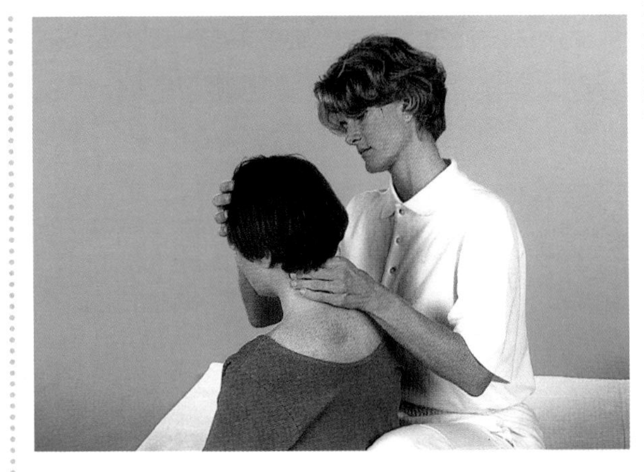

Above: Calm, reassuring holds will enable your partner to relax tense muscles.

Use relaxing music to calm yourself and your partner; soft, rather than bright, lighting will create the right atmosphere. Avoid eating for two hours before the treatment and wear comfortable clothing, preferably pure cotton.

Effects of the Treatment

The immediate effect of Shiatsu treatment is individual. A sense of well-being is common. The time factor in the relief of symptoms depends on the nature of the condition. Because of the deep relaxation that usually occurs and the stimulus to the major body systems, your partner may experience "healing reaction"; flu-like symptoms, aches, changes in bowel movements and urination, headaches or low energy may appear for around 24 hours. These are signs of elimination and show that the healing process is beginning.

Preparation

▶ Before starting your treatment, always take a few moments to prepare yourself and your partner. Sitting in the Seiza position (on your knees) on your partner's right side, place your hand on the sacrum. Sit quietly, regulate your breathing, empty your mind, and focus on how your partner feels to you right now.

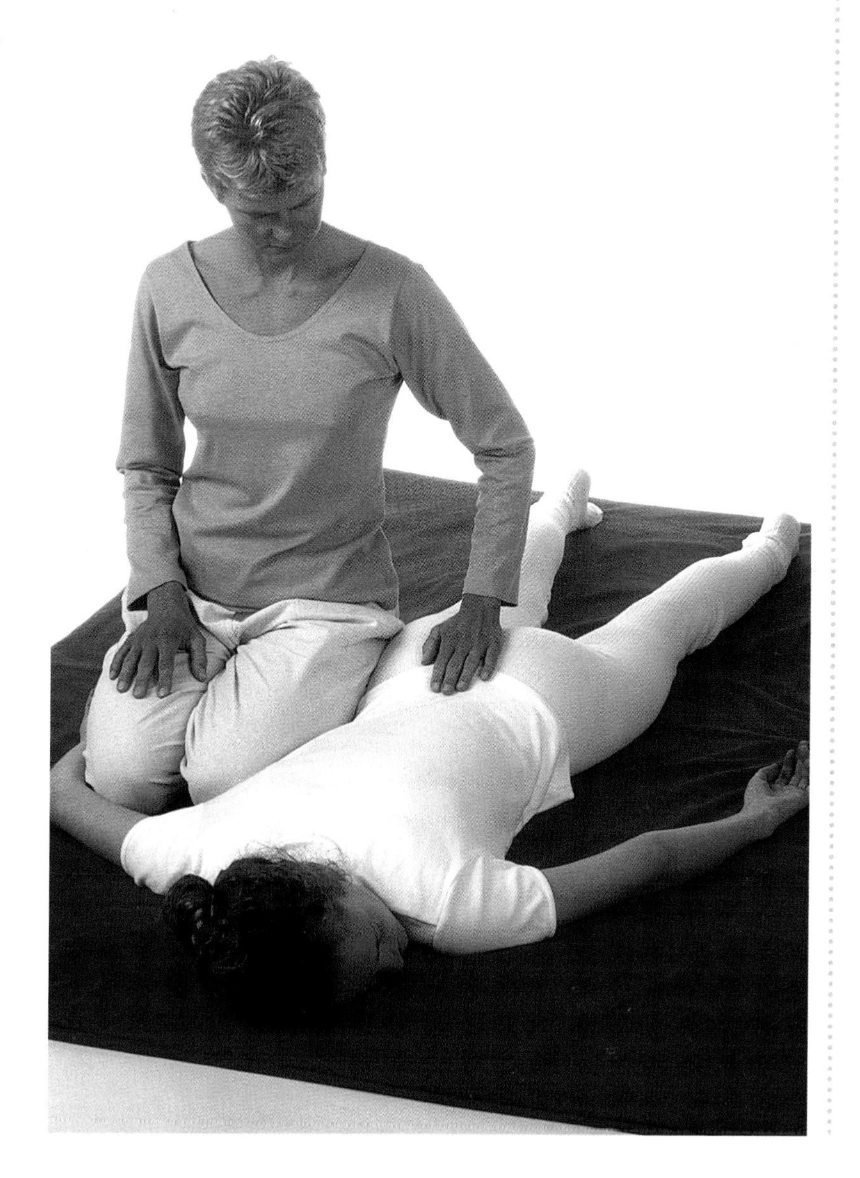

DoIn Exercises

The term "DoIn" literally means "self-massage" and involves a combination of different techniques to improve the circulation and flow of Ki throughout the whole body.

The following exercises can be used not only to revitalize tired muscles and low spirits, but also to relieve a stiff, tensed body and a stressed mind. Starting your day with a DoIn session will awaken your body and mind and help you feel refreshed and ready for the coming day. Repeating the routine in the evening before you go to bed will be physically and mentally relaxing and encourage a deep, peaceful night's sleep. Keep a natural posture and breathing throughout the exercises and try to maintain an empty mind, free from any disturbing thoughts and feelings.

Preparation

▶ Prepare yourself by gently shaking out your body. Shake your arms and hands to help release any tension in your upper body. Gently shake out your legs and feet as well. Place your feet shoulder-width apart and unlock your knees. Straighten your back to allow better energy flow, relax your shoulders and close your eyes. Take a minute to focus internally and get in touch with how you and your body feel before starting the DoIn routine. Become aware of any areas that might be in discomfort and try to empty your mind of disturbing or distracting thoughts.

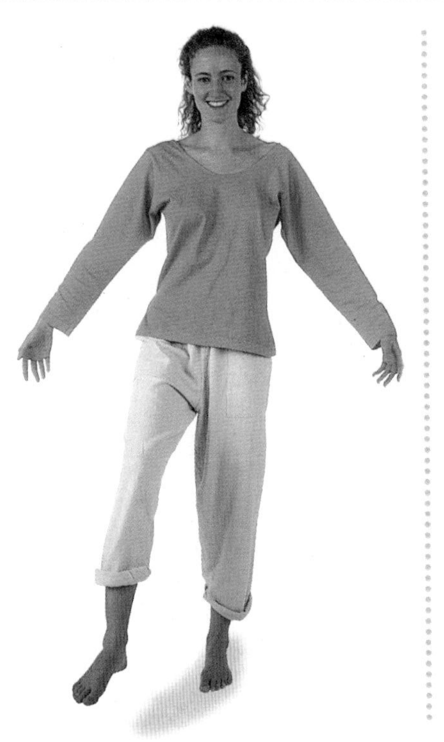

Head and Face

1

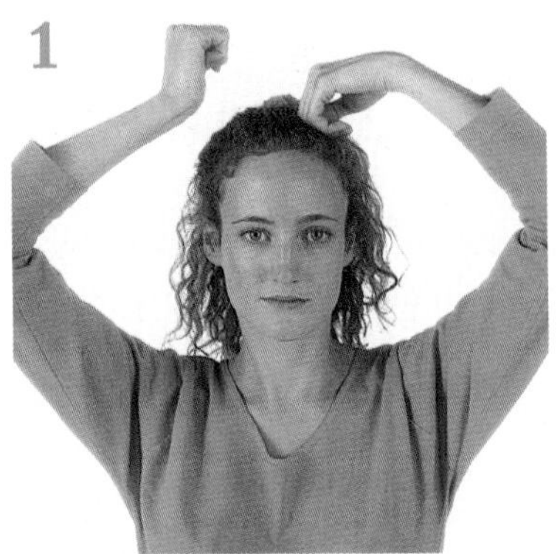

▲ Open your eyes and make a loose fist with both hands. Keep your wrists relaxed and gently start to tap the top of your head.

2

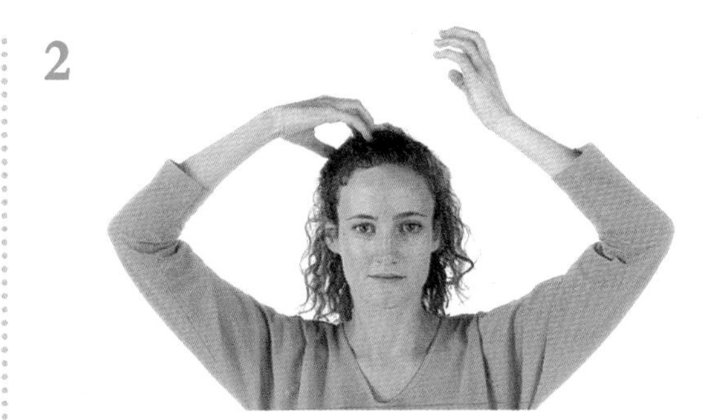

▲ Adjust the percussion pressure as needed and use your fingertips or the palm of your hand for lighter stimulation. Slowly work your way all around the head, covering the sides, front and back. This exercise will wake up your brain and stimulate blood circulation, which will be beneficial for your mental focus and concentration as well as the quality of your hair.

3

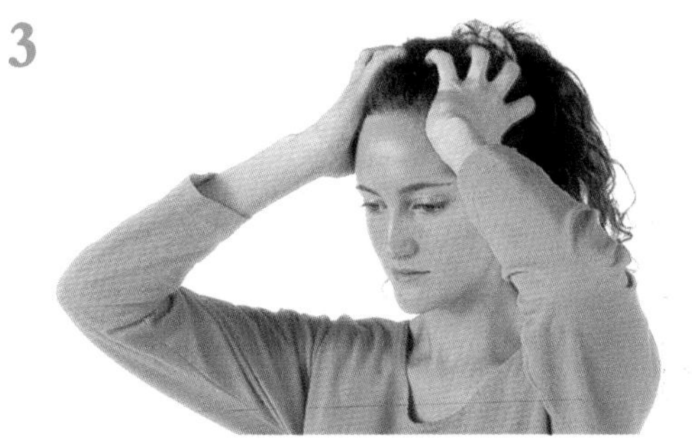

▲ Pull your fingers through your hair a few times, stimulating the Bladder and Gall Bladder meridians running across the top and side of your head.

4

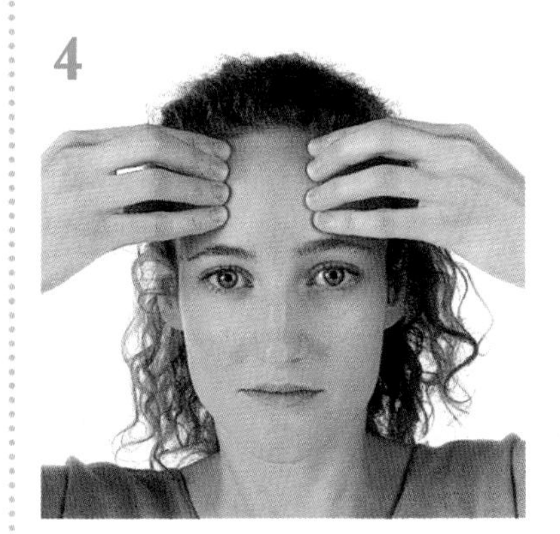

▲ Place your fingers on your forehead, apply a little pressure and stroke outwards from the centre to the temples. Repeat this three times.

5

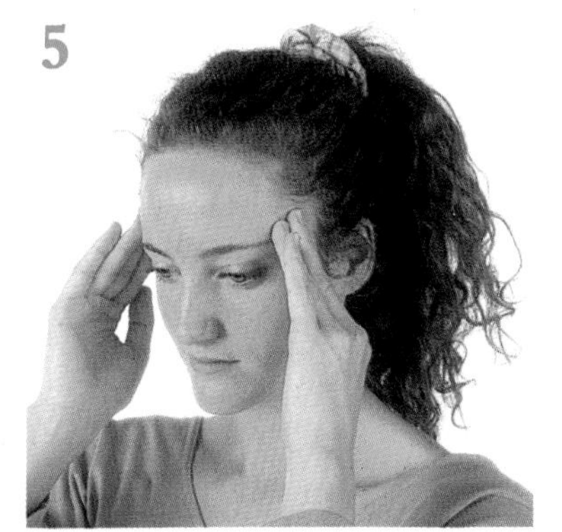

▲ Bring your fingers to your temples. Drop your elbows, relax your shoulders and gently massage your temples, using small circular movements. This can prevent and relieve headaches.

6

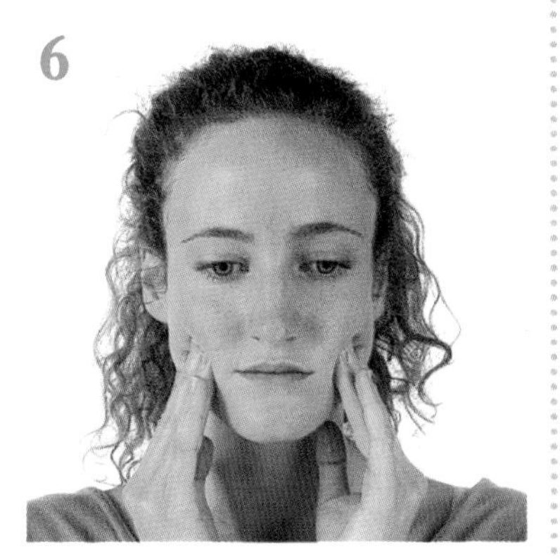

▲ Massage down the sides of your face to the jaw.

7

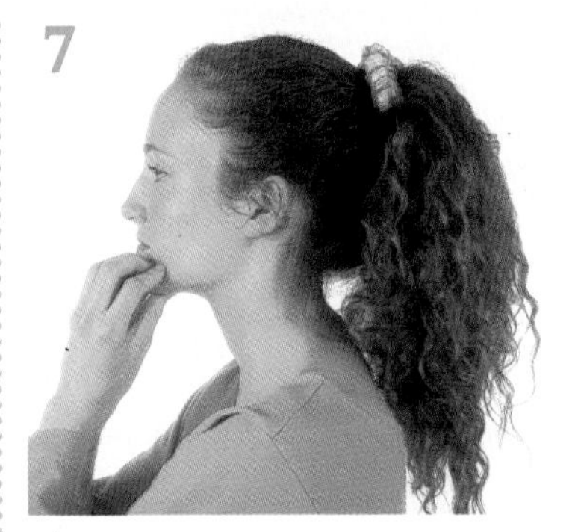

▲ Squeeze along the jawbone, working outwards from the centre. This is a very good technique for relaxation and for stimulating the saliva glands.

8

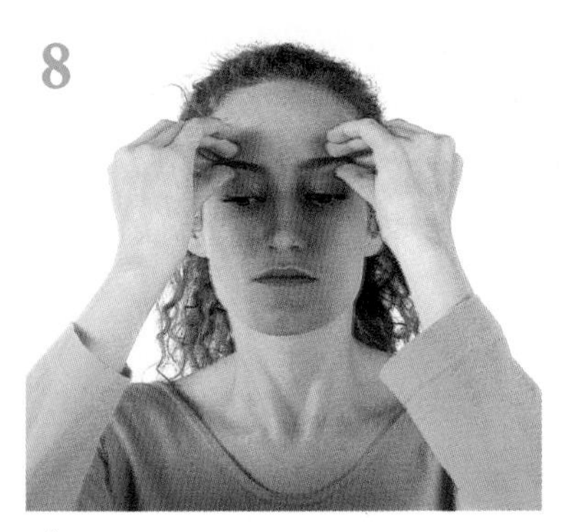

▲ Using your index finger and thumb, squeeze your eyebrows starting from the centre line and moving laterally, three times.

9

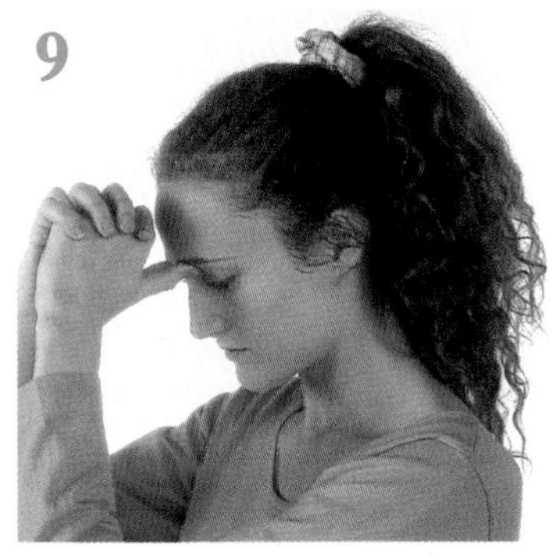

▲ Bring your thumbs to the inside of the eyebrows (point BL2). Allow the weight of your head to rest on your thumbs, stimulating BL2. This helps clear headaches and ease sinus problems.

10

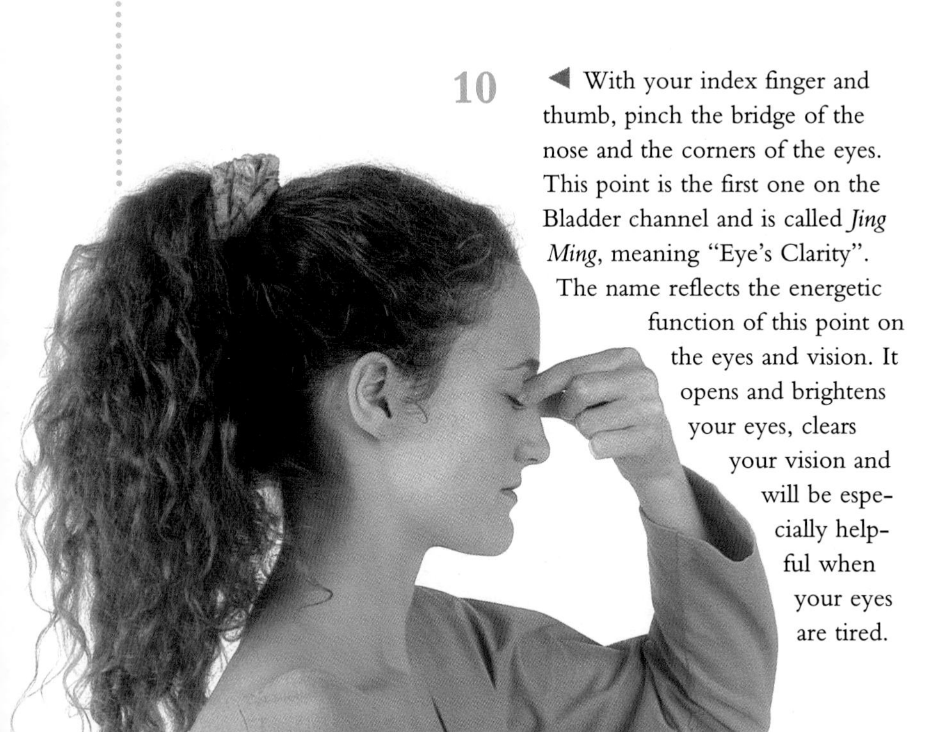

◀ With your index finger and thumb, pinch the bridge of the nose and the corners of the eyes. This point is the first one on the Bladder channel and is called *Jing Ming*, meaning "Eye's Clarity". The name reflects the energetic function of this point on the eyes and vision. It opens and brightens your eyes, clears your vision and will be especially helpful when your eyes are tired.

11

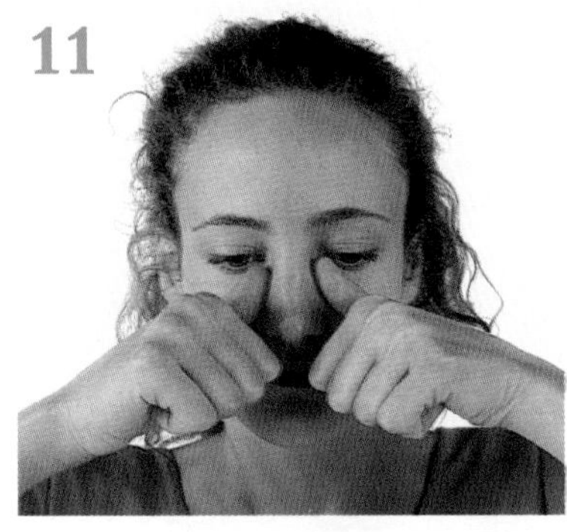

▲ Clench your fingers and apply your thumbs to the sides of your nose. Breathe in as you quickly stroke down the side of your nose. This will help clear your sinuses and release any nasal congestion. Repeat three times.

Neck

1

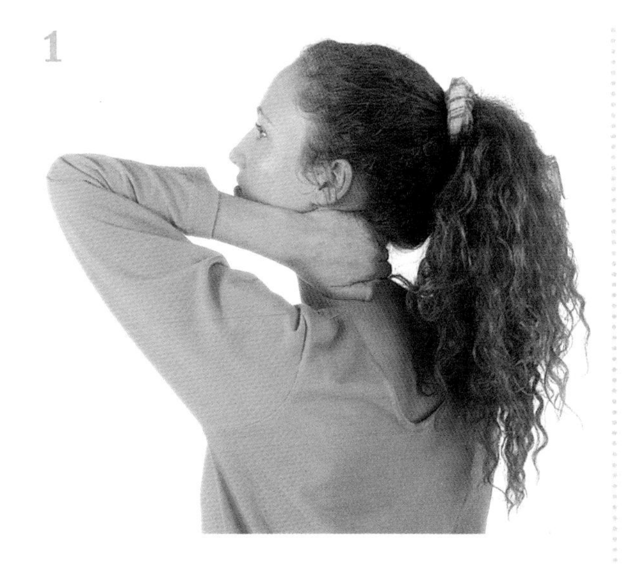

▶ Using one hand, place the palm across the back of your neck and firmly massage in a squeezing motion. This will increase the flow of blood and Ki to the area, release stagnation and remove waste products, such as lactic acid.

2

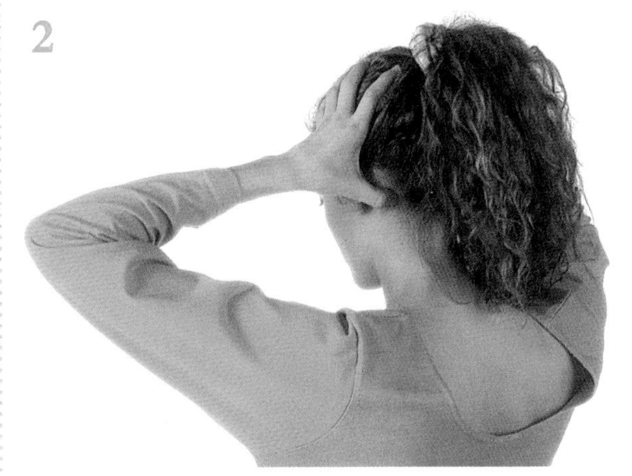

▲ With your thumbs, apply pressure to the point at the base of the skull, directing the pressure upwards against the skull.

3

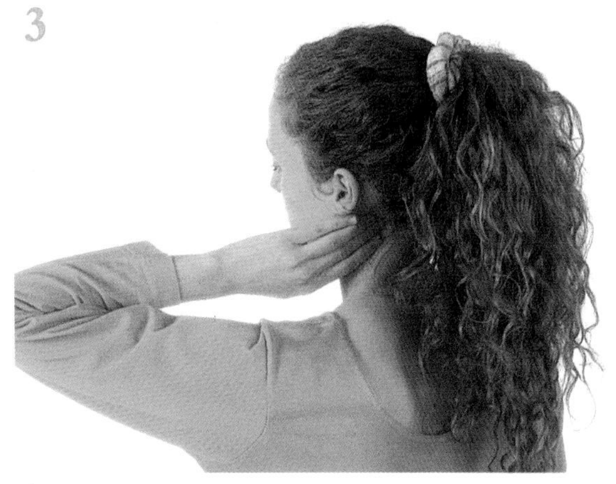

▲ Use your fingers and rub across the muscle fibres at the base of the skull. This will release the muscles and tendons in the area and help relieve headaches and shoulder pain.

Shoulders, Arms and Hands

After doing these exercises shake out your arms. Allow them to relax and compare the feeling in them. Your right arm probably feels lighter, more vital and expanded compared to the left. This shows that there is a better energy flow in your right arm. Repeat the same techniques on your left arm and hand and then compare them again.

1

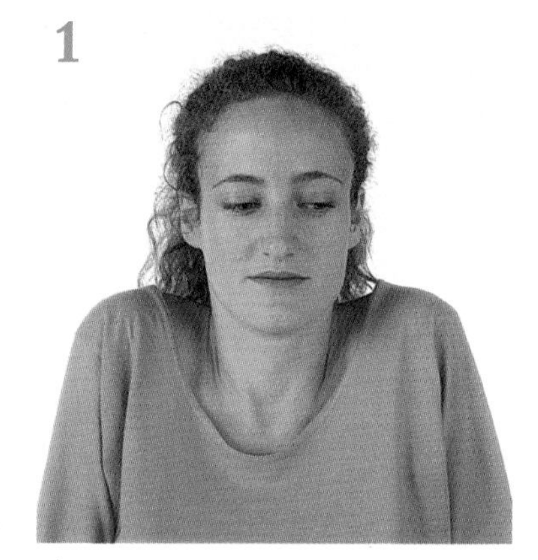

▲ Lift your shoulders up and breathe in. Breathe out, letting your shoulders drop and relax. Repeat.

2

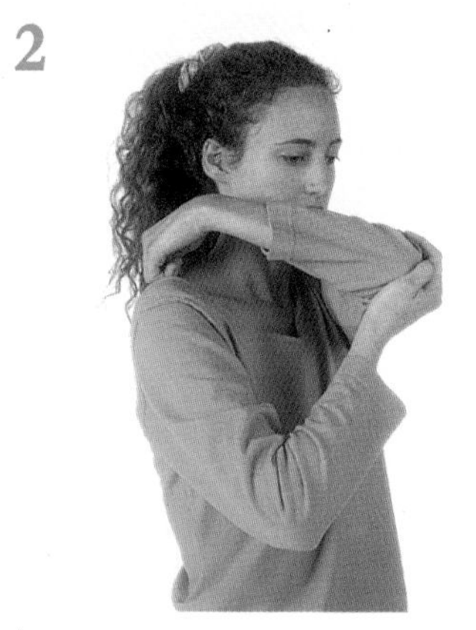

▲ Support your left elbow and with a loose fist tap across your shoulder.

3

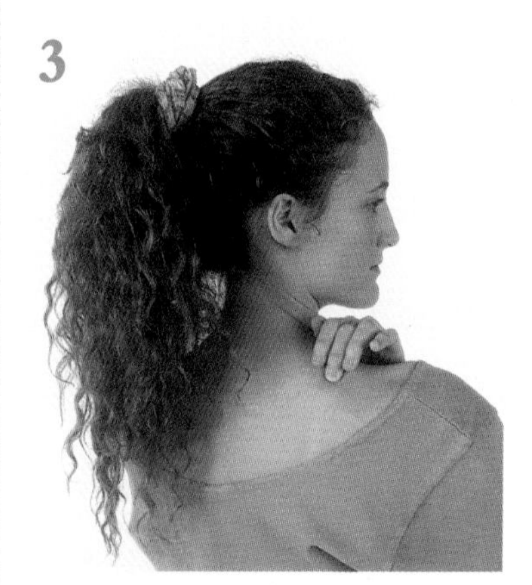

▲ Press your middle finger into the shoulder's highest point, known as point GBL21, "Shoulder Well".

Caution *Do not use in pregnancy.*

4

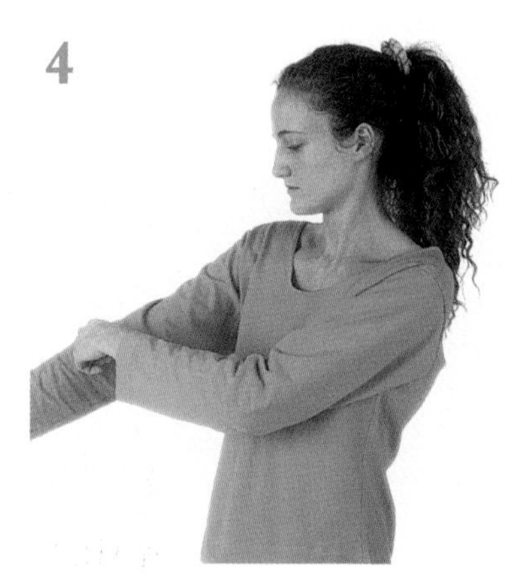

▲ Straighten your arm, open your palm and tap down the inside of your arm from the shoulder to the open hand. This stimulates the energy flow of the Lung, Heart Governor and Heart meridians.

5

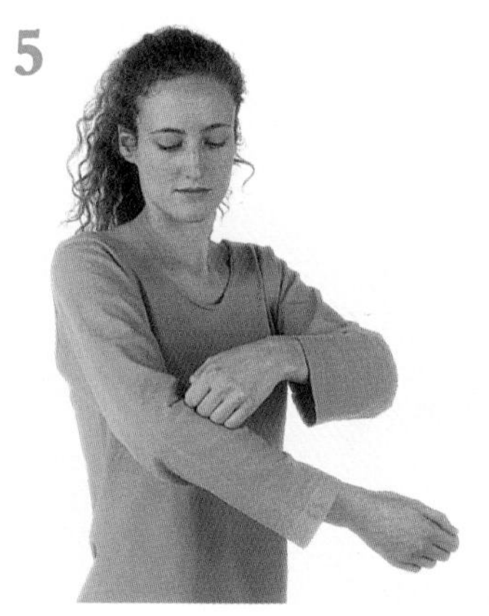

▲ Turn your arm over and tap up the back of your arm, from the hand to the shoulders. This stimulates the meridians for the Large Intestine, Triple Heater and Small Intestine. Repeat three times.

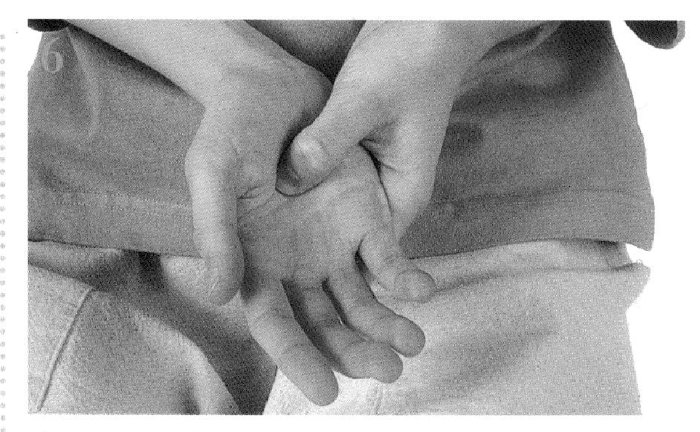

▲ Use your left thumb to work through your right hand, gently massaging the centre of your palm to stimulate the point there, HG8, also known as "Palace of Anxiety". This will relieve general tension and revitalize you physically, mentally and spiritually.

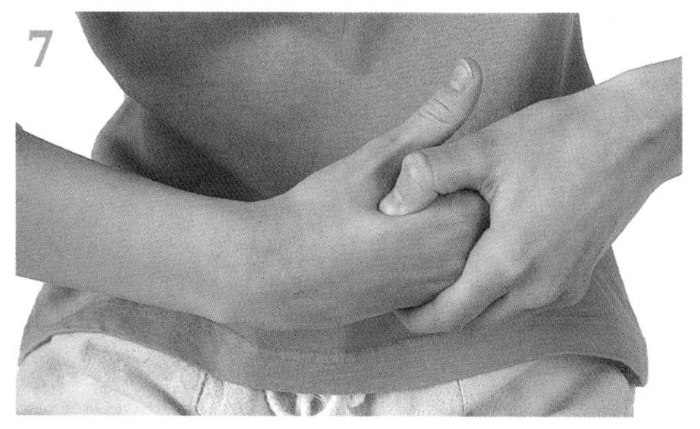

▲ Stimulating "Great Eliminator" on the Large Intestine meridian, in the web between the index finger and the thumb, will help relieve headaches and can also be used to treat constipation or diarrhoea. Good for general health and well-being.

Caution *Sometimes used in childbirth to speed up labour; do not use during pregnancy.*

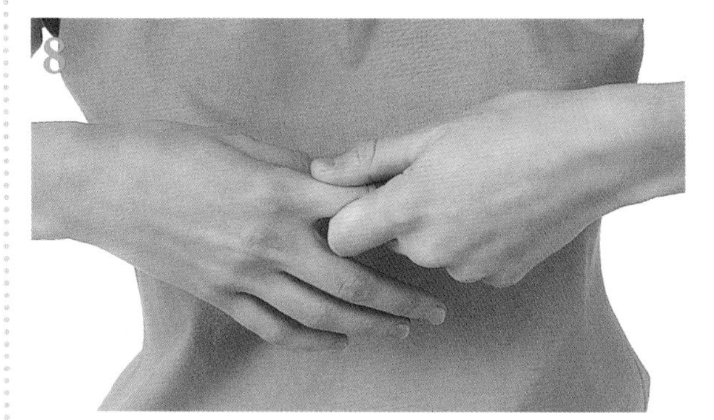

▲ Squeeze and massage the joints of each finger using your index finger and thumb.

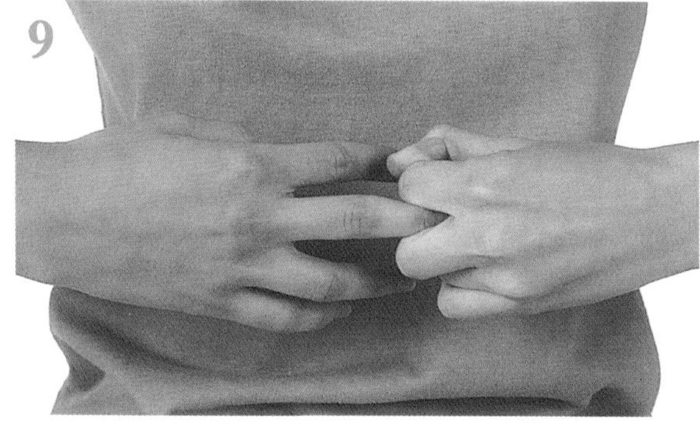

▲ Pulling out the fingers will stimulate the starting and end points of all the meridians. This is a great way to release any stress and tension in your hands and will help prevent arthritis as well as improve flexibility in the joints.

Chest, Abdomen and Lower Back

▶ Open up your chest, and using either a loose fist or flat hands for comfort, tap across your chest, above and around the breasts and across your ribs. This will stimulate your lungs, enhance and strengthen your respiratory system and improve your Blood and Ki circulation. Children love this exercise. It is wonderful for releasing tension in your chest, usually brings a smile to your face and will support you in expressing your inner thoughts and feelings.

1

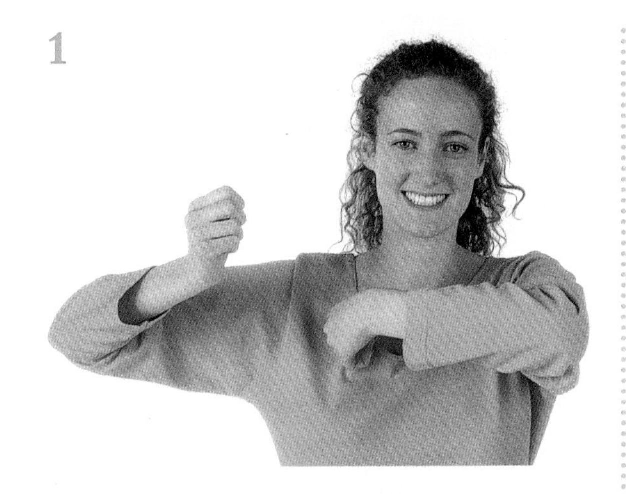

2

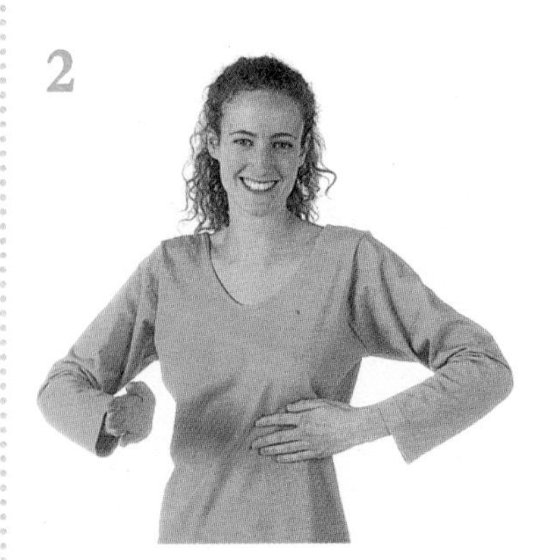

▲ Take a deep breath in as you open your chest again; on the out breath tap your chest and make an "Ahhh…" sound.

3

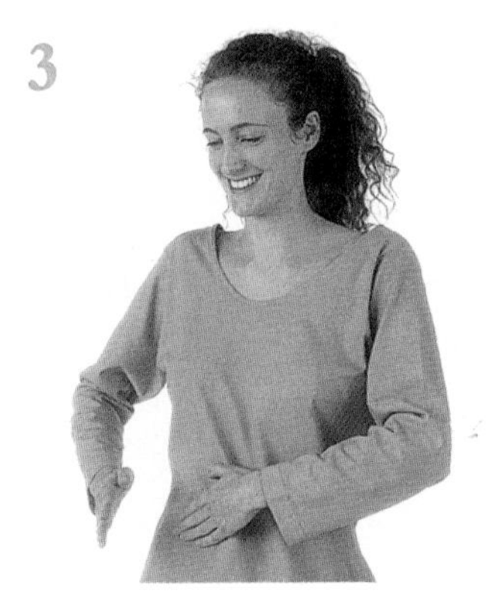

▲ Proceed further down towards your abdomen, and with open hands gently tap around your abdomen in a clockwise direction, moving down on the left side and up on the right. This follows the flow of circulation and digestion. Do this for about a minute.

4

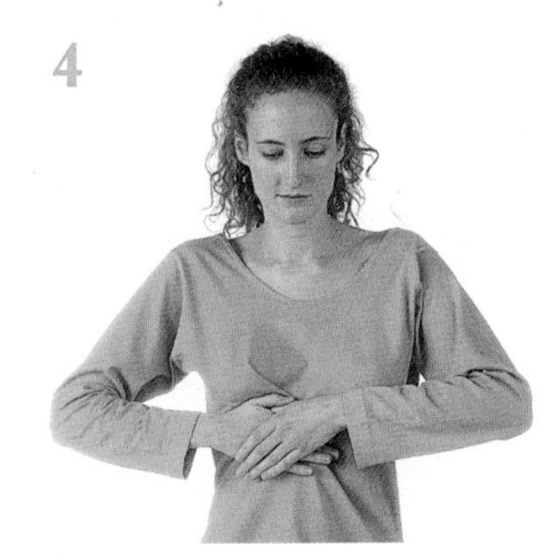

▲ Place one hand on top of the other and make the same circular motion around your abdomen for another minute.

5

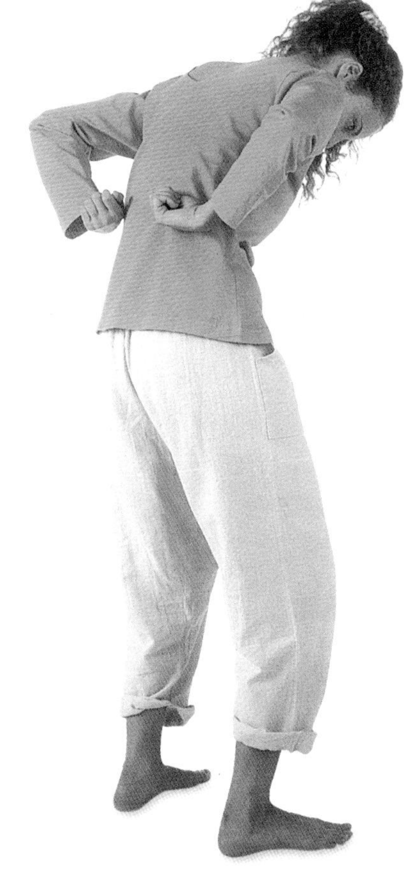

▲ Place your hands on your back, just below your ribcage. This is the area of your kidneys. Start to rub the area until you feel some warmth building up underneath your hands and then proceed to tap the area gently using a loose fist. This will stimulate your Kidney energy responsible for your vitality and also for warming your body.

6

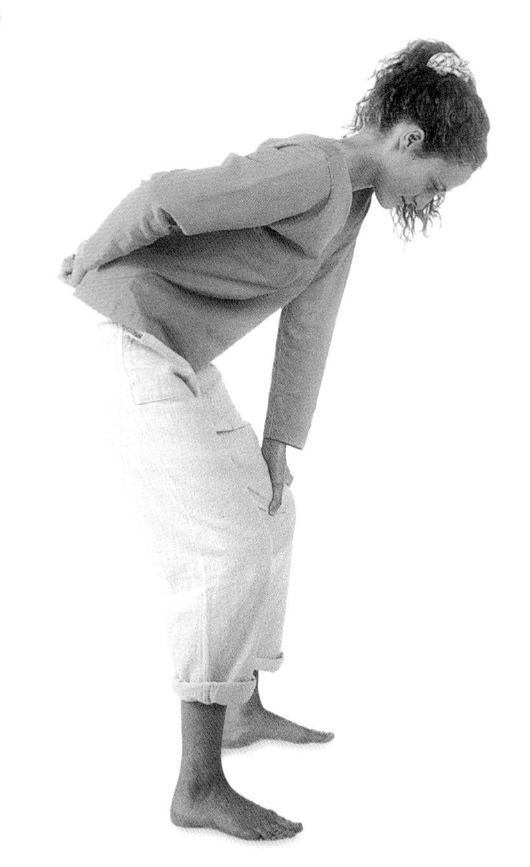

▲ Lean forward and place one hand on your knee. Using the back of your other hand, tap across the sacrum bone at the base of your spine. This will activate your nervous system and send energy vibrations up the spine to your head and brain, bringing clarity to your mental processes.

LEGS

Proceed from the sacrum to your hips and buttocks. Tapping this area will help release muscle tension and stimulate your digestive and elimination organs.

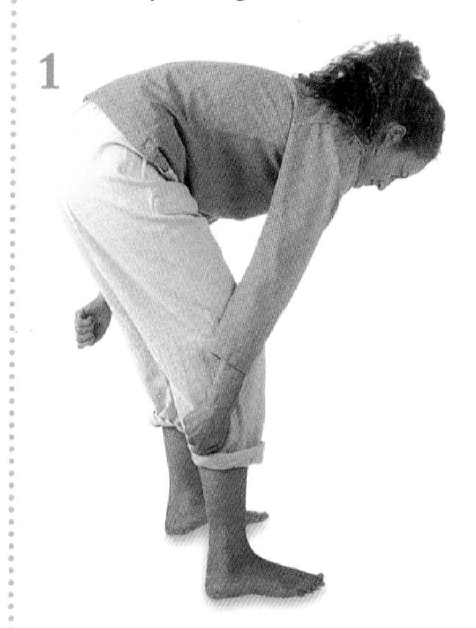

1

▲ Open your feet a bit wider, keep your knees slightly bent and tap down the backs of your legs from your buttocks to your heels, following the flow of energy in your Bladder meridian.

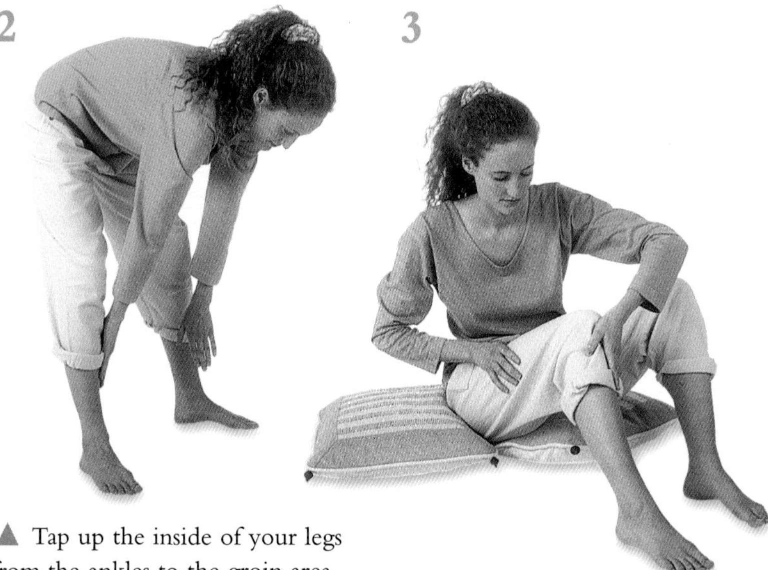

2

▲ Tap up the inside of your legs from the ankles to the groin area, stimulating your Liver and Spleen meridians. Tap down the outside of your legs to stimulate your Gall Bladder meridian and come up the inside of your legs again. Finally tap down the fronts of your legs, slightly outside the big quadriceps muscle, activating your Stomach meridian. Tap all the way down to the fronts of your ankles and then come back up the inside of your legs.

3

▲ Find the point ST36 on the Stomach meridian on the outside of your leg, along the tibia bone. To locate ST36, sit down on the floor, and measure four finger widths down from the patella (knee-cap), place your thumb on the point and apply pressure. ST36 is a good point for general well-being and tired legs.

Feet

1

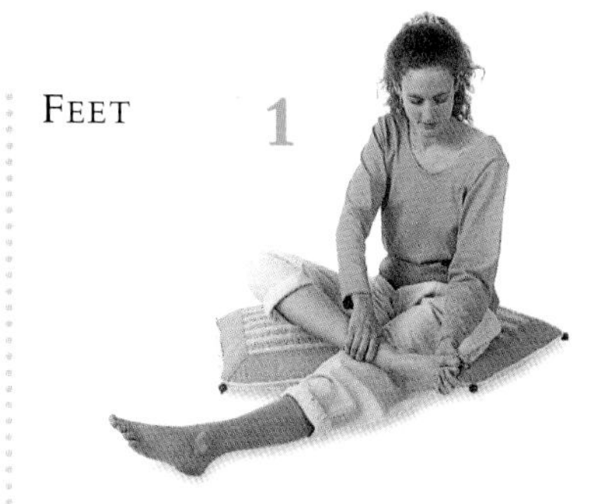

▲ Sit on the floor, take your right foot in your hands and circle it from the ankle to mobilize the joint generally.

▼ On the dorsal part of your foot, between the big toe and the second toe is LIV3, "Big Rush". A very good point to stimulate if you experience abdominal spasm and cramps.

Caution *Do not use this point during pregnancy.*

2

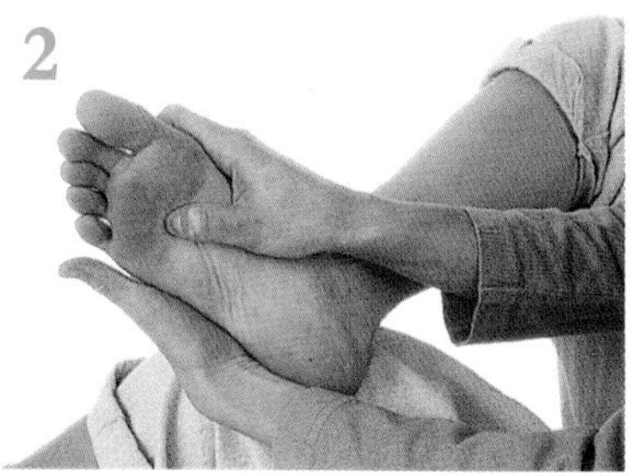

▲ Massage the sole of your foot using your thumbs. About one-third of the distance from the base of the second toe to the back of your heel, you will find KID1, "Gushing Spring". The name suggests this point's fresh and active energy and stimulating it with pressure will have a revitalizing effect upon your whole system. Give the whole foot an invigorating rub.

3

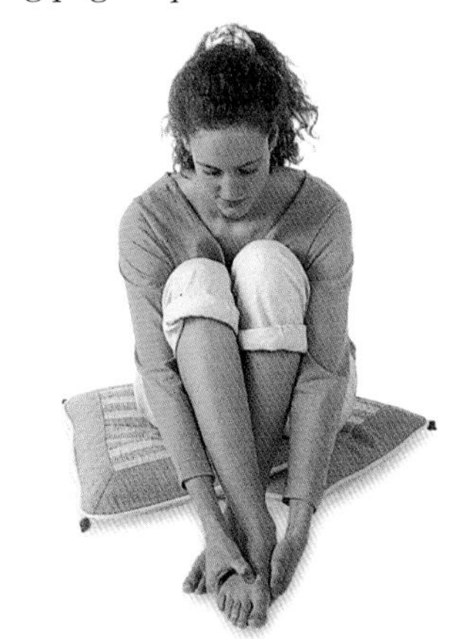

► Take hold of your ankle with both hands and shake out your foot. Repeat the same sequence with your left foot.

4

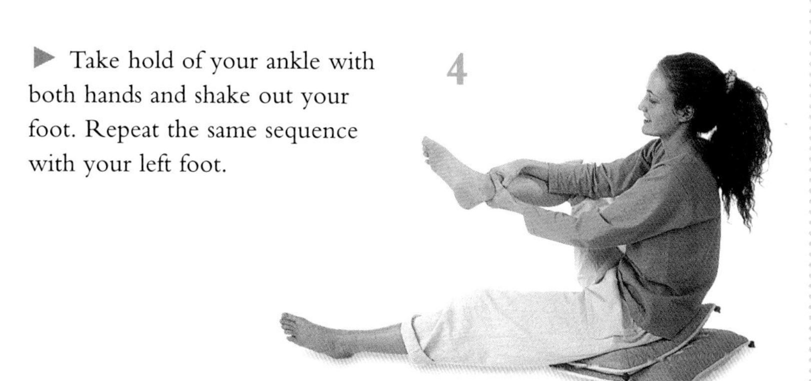

Completion

After having worked through your whole body, stand up and gently shake out again. Place your feet shoulder-width apart and bend your knees slightly. Imagine a string through your spine, from the tail bone to the top of your head. Stretch the string and feel your spine straighten up to allow for better Ki flow. Close your eyes for a moment and see how you feel after your DoIn session. Try to remember how you felt at the beginning and compare that with the sensation you have now.

Open your eyes again and to complete your session, practise the breathing exercise.

Breathing to Calm the Mind

This "Qi Gong" breathing exercise will calm your mind, bring your energy down to the lower body, and you will feel centred in your *Hara* (belly) afterwards. Breathe in through your nose and out through your mouth throughout the sequence and focus your breath in your lower abdomen.

1

◀ Remain in the same standing position as for the DoIn exercises and make a nice rounded shape with your arms, bringing your hands together in front of your navel. Allow the palms to face up to the ceiling.

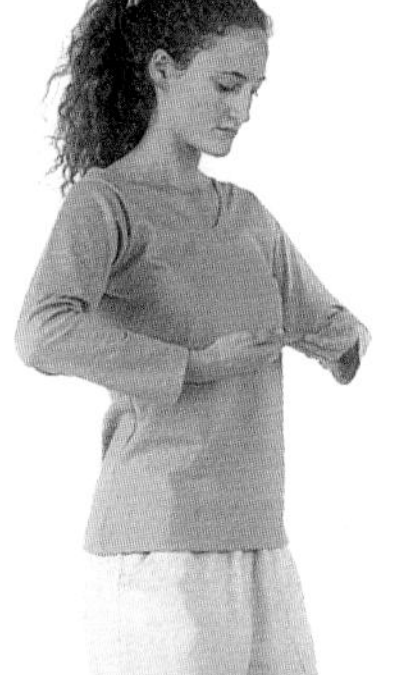

2

▶ Slowly lift your hands up towards your solar plexus area as you breathe in.

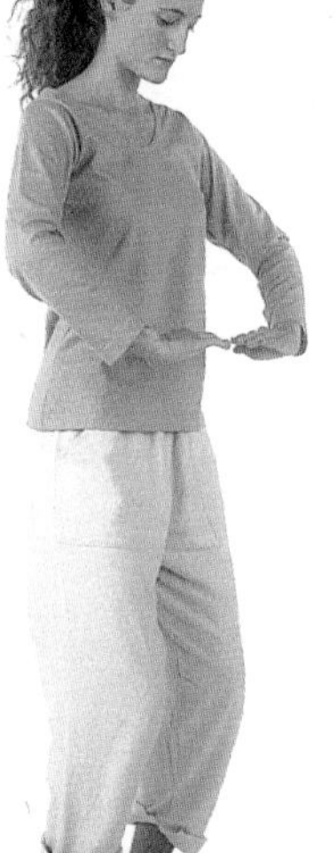

3

◀ Turn your palms to the floor and press down towards the floor, straightening your arms slowly as you breathe out.

▶ Breathe in again and bring your hands back to your solar plexus area.

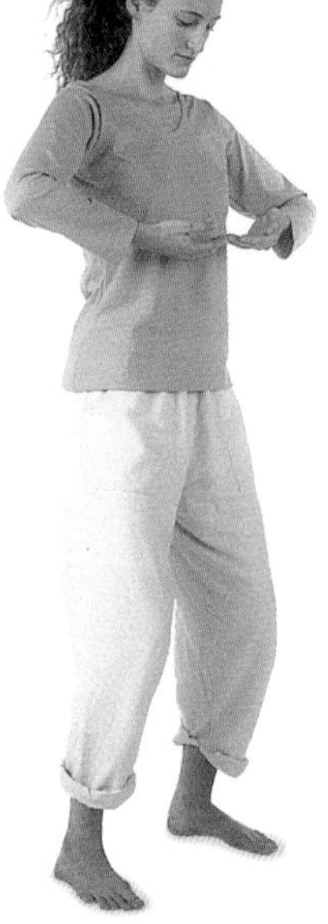

4

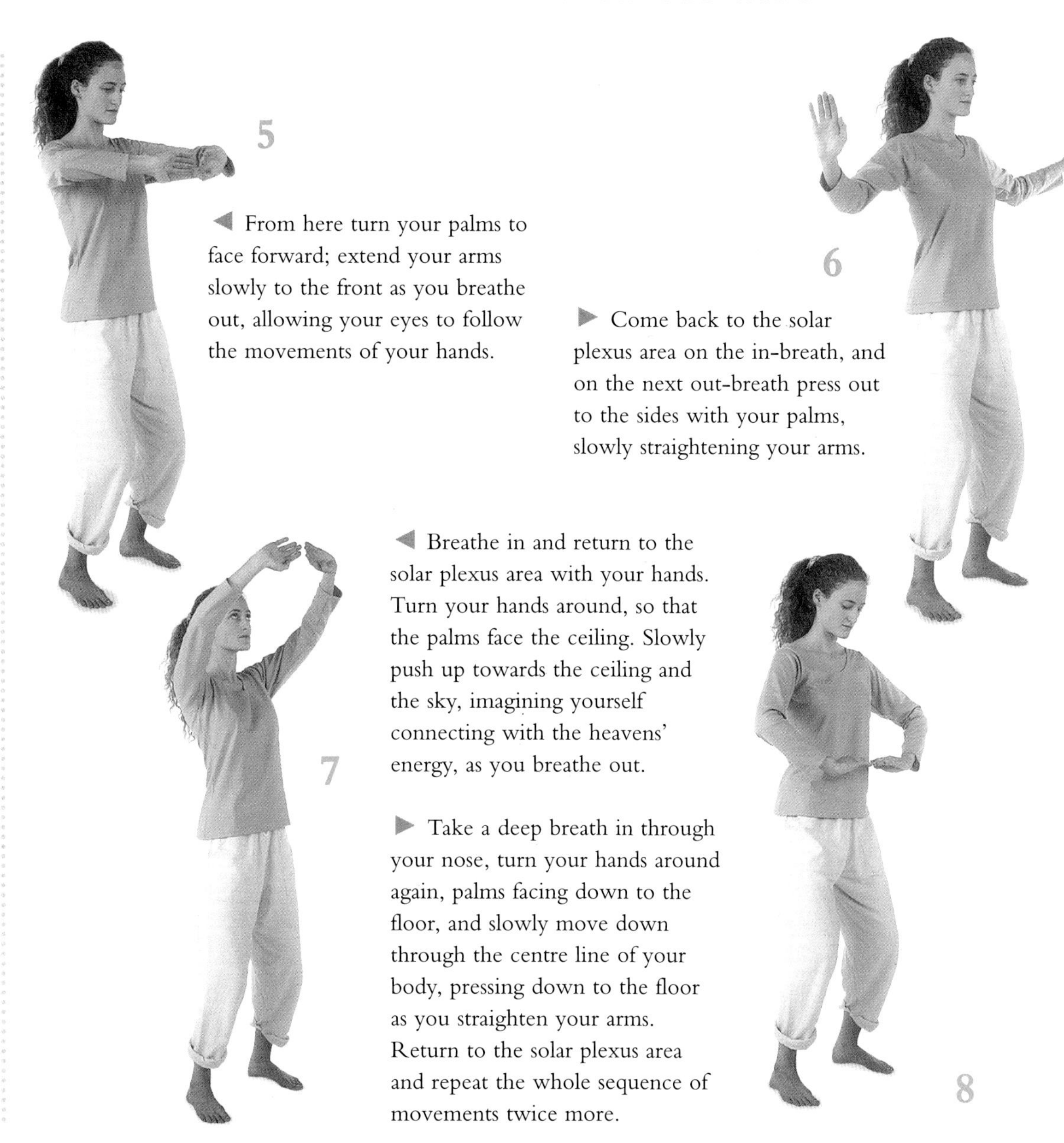

5

◀ From here turn your palms to face forward; extend your arms slowly to the front as you breathe out, allowing your eyes to follow the movements of your hands.

6

▶ Come back to the solar plexus area on the in-breath, and on the next out-breath press out to the sides with your palms, slowly straightening your arms.

7

◀ Breathe in and return to the solar plexus area with your hands. Turn your hands around, so that the palms face the ceiling. Slowly push up towards the ceiling and the sky, imagining yourself connecting with the heavens' energy, as you breathe out.

8

▶ Take a deep breath in through your nose, turn your hands around again, palms facing down to the floor, and slowly move down through the centre line of your body, pressing down to the floor as you straighten your arms. Return to the solar plexus area and repeat the whole sequence of movements twice more.

Nervous System Calmers: Self Help

Stress can have a dramatic effect on the nervous system and badly affects body functions such as breathing, digestion, circulation and hormonal regulation. Balancing the energy in the Bladder channel through the following back exercises and Shiatsu treatment of the back will have a calming effect on the nervous system. The following exercises will gently work through your whole spine, easing up blockages and improving flexibility and energy movements throughout. While performing the different exercises, you might find that some areas are more tense and uncomfortable than others. Pay attention to these specific areas and use your breathing to ease any pain.

Swinging the Arms

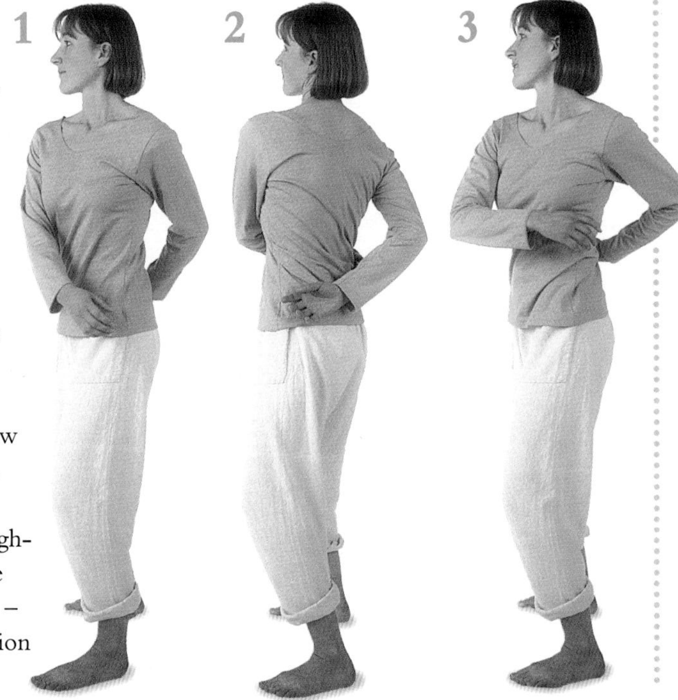

- Stand with your feet shoulder-width apart and knees slightly bent. Keep your back straight. Allow your arms to hang loose at your sides. Slowly start swinging your arms from side to side, keeping them at waist level.

- Swinging your arms will create a twist in your spine, loosening up the joints between the lumbar vertebrae and allowing for better and more flexible movement.

- Bring your arms a bit higher up so that you now feel the twist in the middle part of your back. This will loosen up the thoracic vertebrae and the diaphragm muscle. If you swing your arms even higher up, level with your shoulders, you will affect the internal organs on this level – your heart and lungs – as you loosen up the upper part of the thoracic region of your spine.

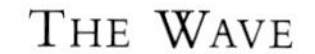

The Wave

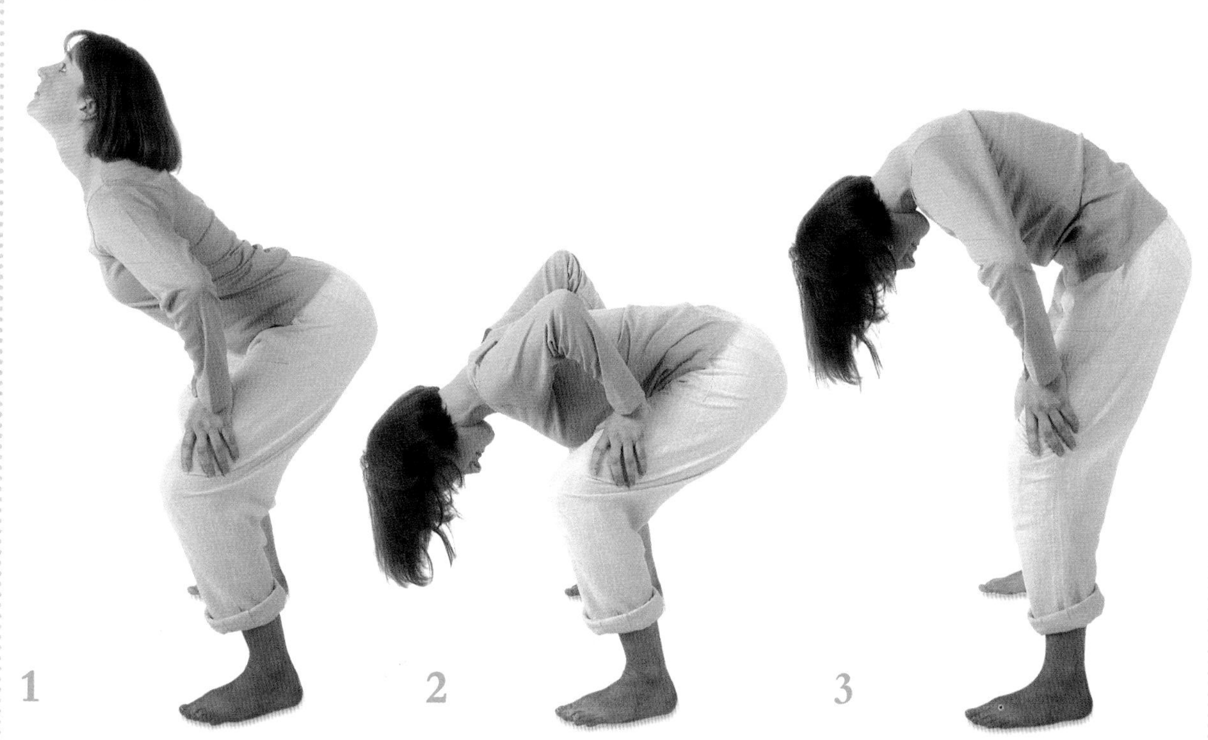

▲ With your feet a bit wider than shoulder-width apart and knees bent, place your hands on your legs, just above your knees, and straighten your back. Sway back and look up to the ceiling.

▲ Bend your arms and slowly bring your upper body down towards the floor, making a deeper squat as you do this. Keep looking up at the ceiling until you can no longer see it. Then relax your head downwards and bring your back into flexion.

▲ Pull your abdominal muscles in and slowly roll up your spine from your sacrum, allowing the head to come up last. Lift your head up and straighten your spine. Move directly into the sway back again and repeat the whole movement about ten times. Imagine a wave rolling up your back, from the base of your spine to the top of your head.

Twisting

1

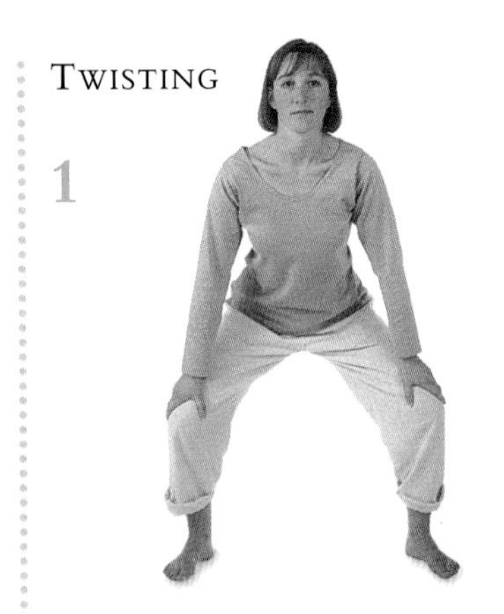

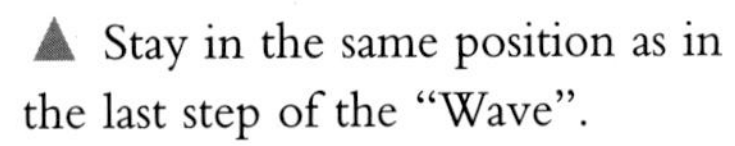

▲ Stay in the same position as in the last step of the "Wave".

2

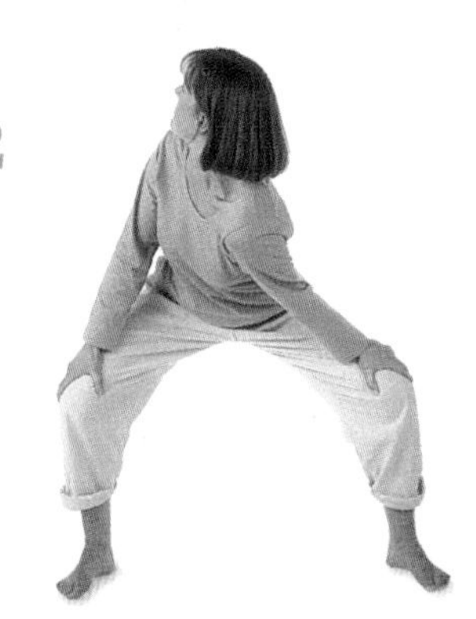

▲ Breathe in and, on the exhalation, drop your left shoulder down as shown. Keep your elbows gently locked and look up to the ceiling over your right shoulder. Feel the twist in your spine.

3

◀ Take another deep breath in, return to the starting position and drop your right shoulder down as you exhale. Repeat another three or four times on each side. Finish by coming back to the starting position. Relax your upper body forward. Move your feet closer together and slowly roll up your spine, until you come to a relaxed standing position.

Relaxation Pose

▼ When you have finished these spinal exercises it is good to lie down on the floor and relax with your lower legs resting on a chair. This relaxes the lumbar area of your back and realigns the whole spine. Close your eyes, allow your breathing to slow down and feel the energy moving from the top of your spine down to the sacrum like a wave. Stay in this position for 10–15 minutes.

This relaxation exercise works directly on the nervous system, calming it down, and you can use the exercise at any time when you feel stressed or when your back is aching after a long day's work.

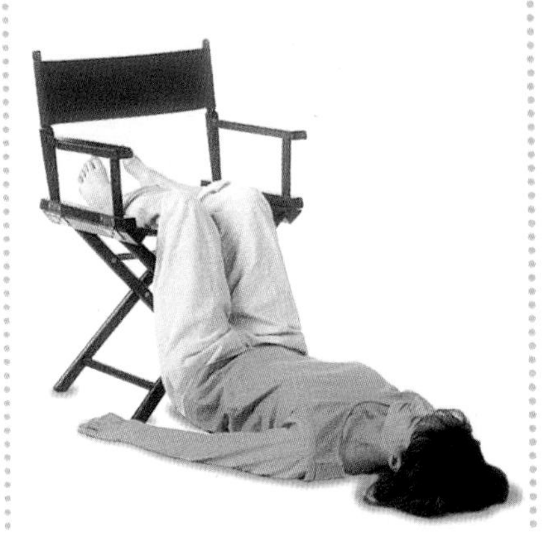

TENNIS BALLS AS EXTRA TOOLS

▶ To treat your back further in case of pain and tension, or whenever you feel in need of general relaxation, try using tennis balls as extra help. Put two tennis balls into a sock and knot the top. Lower yourself on to the tennis balls, which should be placed on either side of the spine. This is where your Bladder meridian is located. Start from the area between your shoulders, or anywhere you feel pain and discomfort.

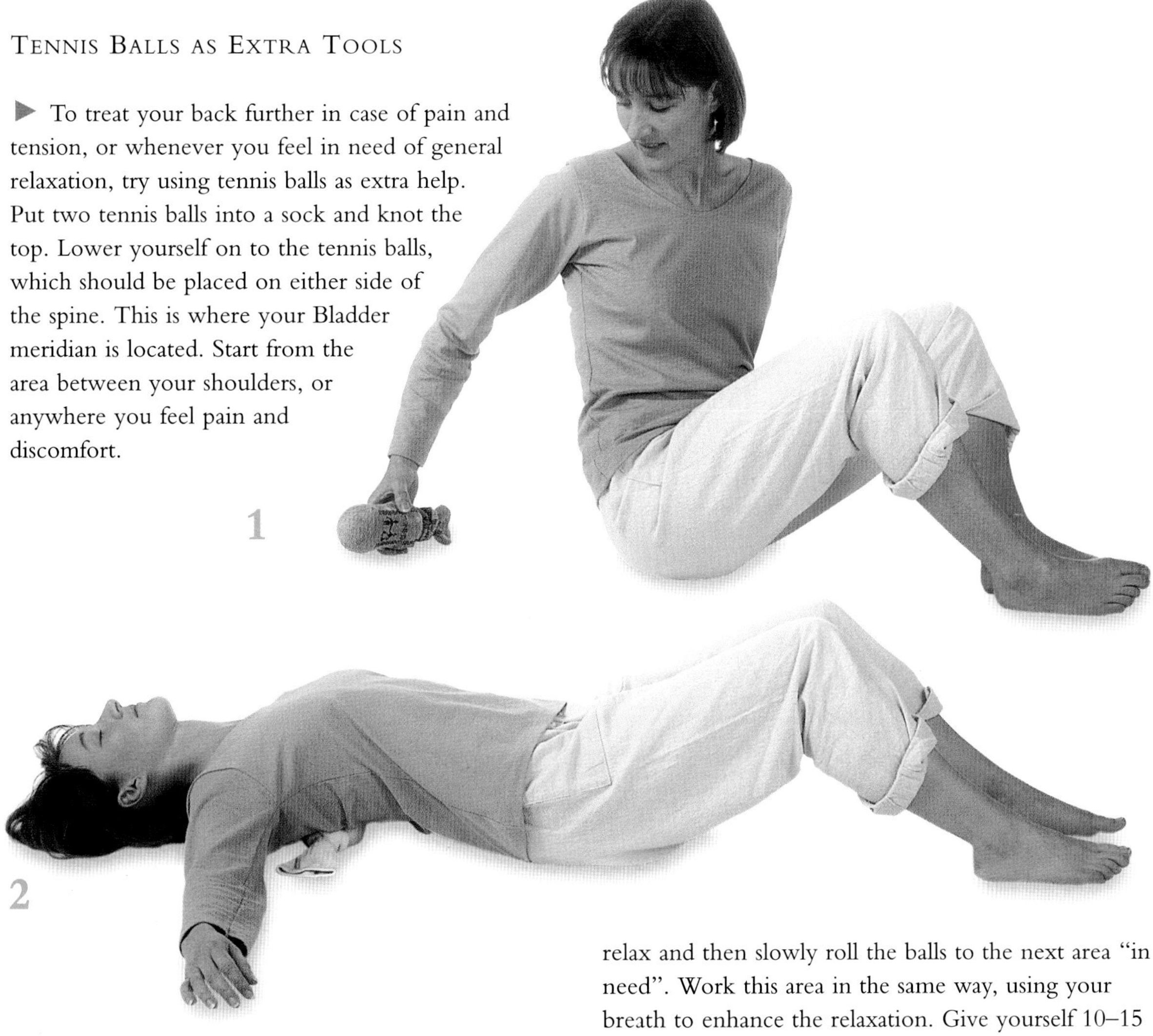

▲ Breathe deeply and allow your back to sink on to the balls. The balls will mould themselves to the contours of your back and stimulate your Bladder energy. Keep the balls in one place until you feel the muscles relax and then slowly roll the balls to the next area "in need". Work this area in the same way, using your breath to enhance the relaxation. Give yourself 10–15 minutes, working down the whole spine. Afterwards your spine will feel open and relaxed against the floor. You will feel calm and have a pleasant sensation of warmth all the way down your back.

Nervous System Calmers: Back Treatment with a Partner

If your partner is feeling tense and stressed, the following Shiatsu techniques will help them to unwind completely and allow your touch to relieve tensions and blocked energy, working on the back to relax and refresh the nervous system. Take time to prepare for the treatment, making sure your partner is comfortable and that you are calm and focused.

Palming Down the Back

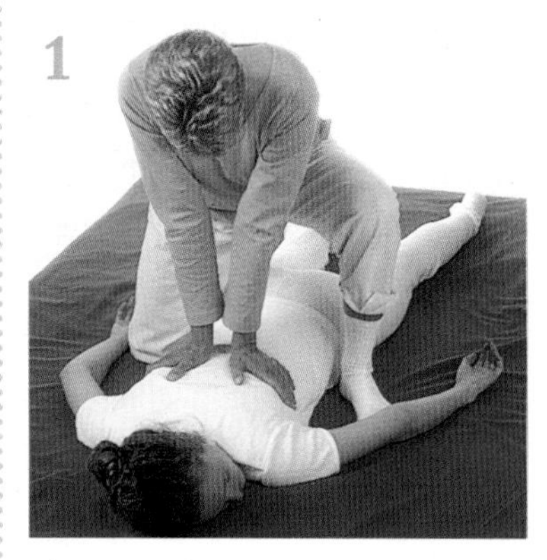

▲ To prepare for treatment, kneel by your partner's side and place your hand at the base of the spine. Concentrate on how your partner feels. Then place your palms on either side of your partner's spine, you may wish to straddle your partner's back.

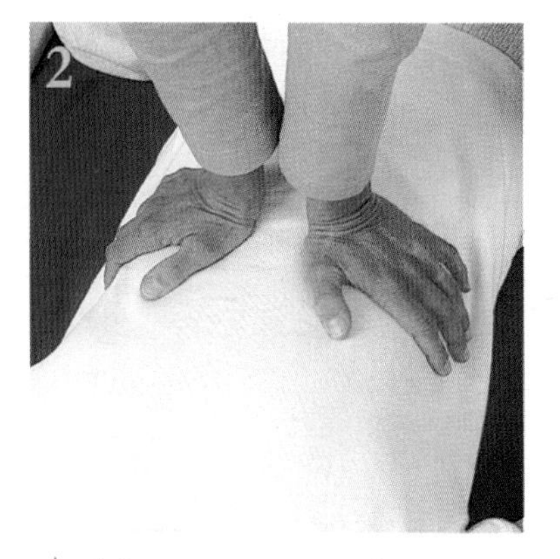

▲ Ask your partner to breathe in; on the out-breath lean into your hands and apply pressure to your partner's back. Ease the pressure applied to allow your partner to breathe in again. Move your hands down and reapply pressure on the next exhalation.

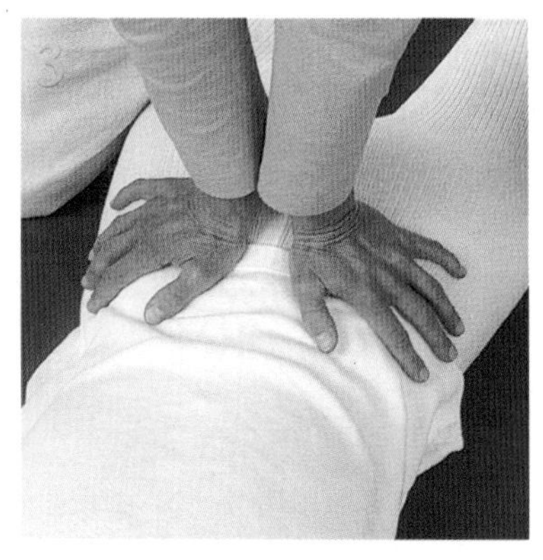

▲ Start at the top of the back between the shoulder-blades. Work your way down to the sacrum. Repeat three times. Keep your elbows straight and use your body weight as you work from your *Hara*.

Rocking the Back

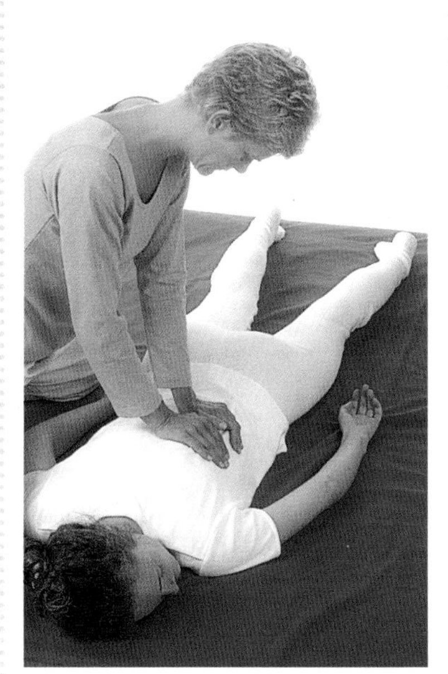

▲ Kneel at 90 degrees to your partner, place your palms in the valley (on the opposite side of the spine) formed by the spinous processes (spinal bumps) and the broad muscles running on either side of the spine. Rock the body with the heels of your hands. As you rock, you can move your hands down the back, one following the other. The rocking should be continuous and rhythmic. Repeat three times. Do both sides, working from the opposite side of the body.

Rocking the Spine

▼ This technique allows you to focus specifically upon the spinal column. You still need to rock; however, this time the spinous processes are gripped between the fingers and the thumbs. Applying a positive (firm) contact, gradually work the hands along the full length of the spine, moving it from side to side. This action loosens the muscles and stimulates the nervous system.

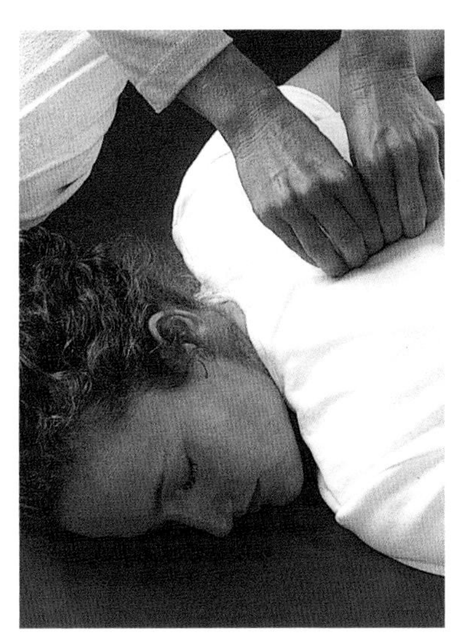

Sawing Action

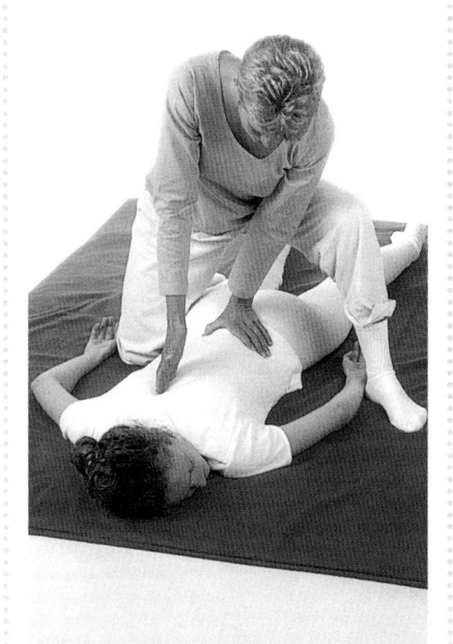

▲ Place your left hand on your partner's sacrum. Using the edge of your right hand like a knife, perform a sawing action down either side of the spine. Work both sides alternately, repeating three times.

Applying Thumb Pressure

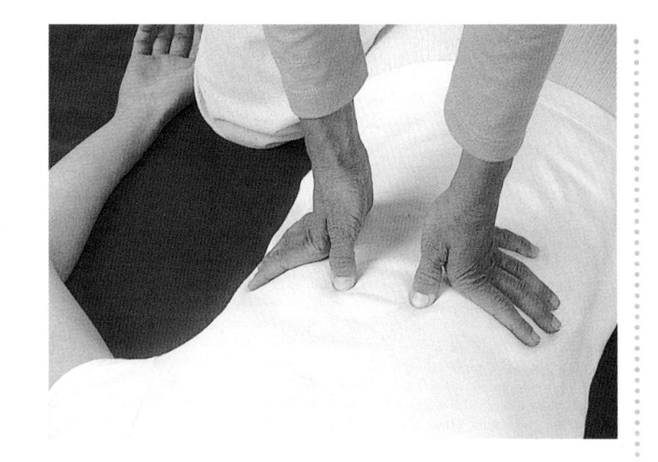

▶ The inner Bladder channel runs the length of the spine, two fingers' breadth on either side of the midline of the spine. Run your hand along the spine and you will feel the undulations of the spinous processes. Bring your thumbs, sideways, two fingers' breadth from the depression between two spinous processes. Apply perpendicular pressure following the breathing of your partner. Start from the top of the back and work down to the sacrum.

Palming the Sacrum

▼ Put one hand on top of the other and place your hands on your partner's sacrum. Apply pressure to the sacrum, focusing the energy into the base of the spine.

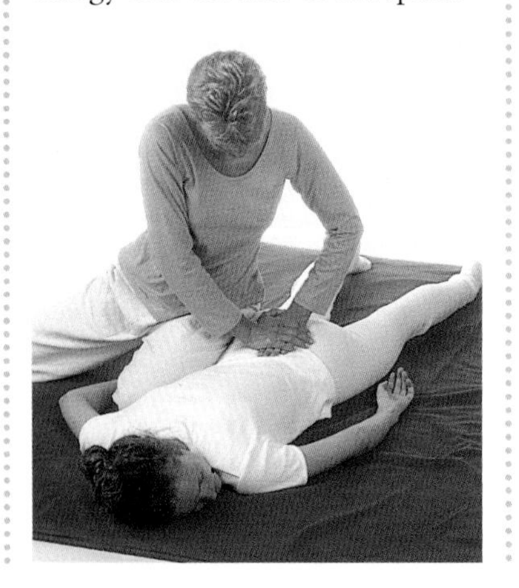

Forearms Across the Buttocks

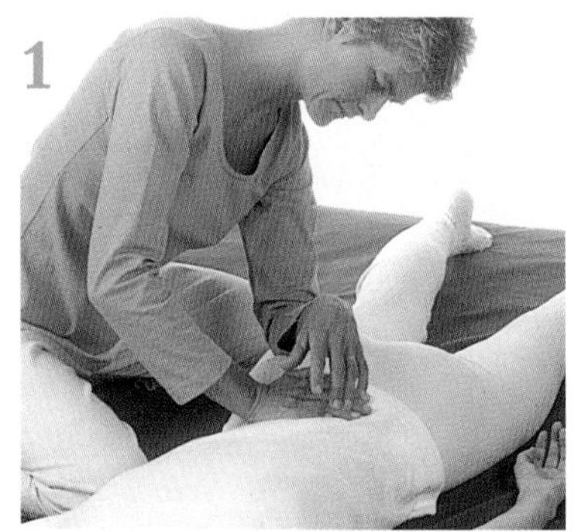

▲ Turn around to face your partner, spread your knees and, using the fleshy part of your forearm in a penetrating and rolling action, apply pressure across the buttocks. You may work both buttocks from the same side of your partner.

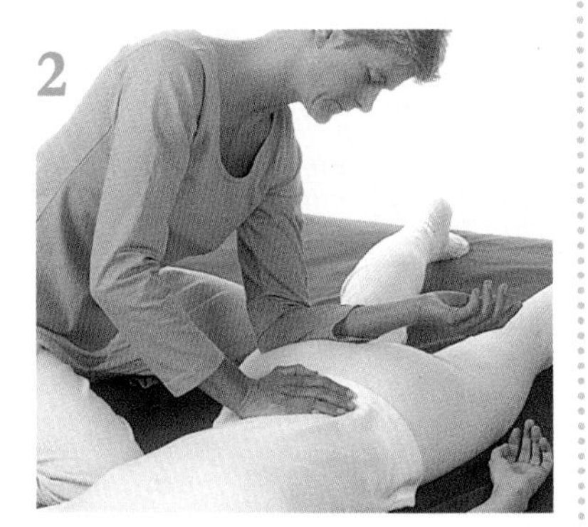

▲ Note the position of the "mother hand" and keep the hands relaxed as you roll your forearm across the buttocks.

Palming the Back of the Leg

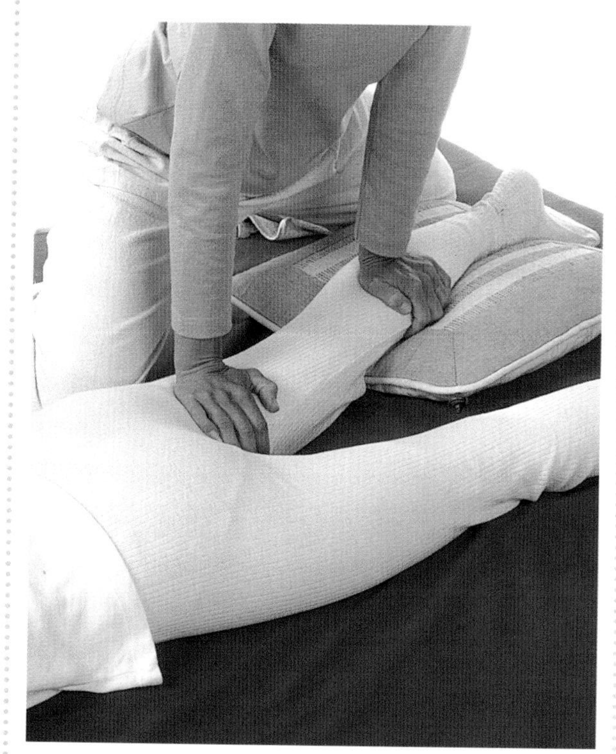

▲ Adjust your position so that you can move down the leg without having to overstretch or become unbalanced. One hand remains on the sacrum. Starting from the back of the thigh, gradually work down the leg, applying pressure with the heel of the hand or your thumb. Support your partner's lower leg with a cushion underneath the shin and be aware of the knee-cap against the floor, i.e. do not apply pressure to the back of the knee. If you feel overstretched, you can move your hand from the sacrum down to the back of the thigh.

Stretching the Ankle to the Buttock

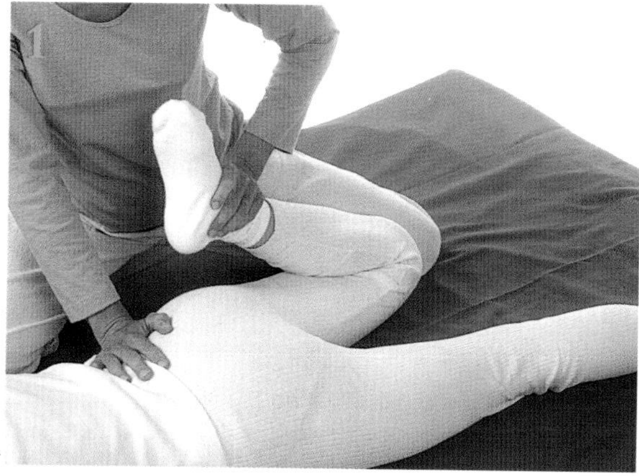

▲ Take hold of your partner's ankle and bend the leg towards the buttock. Adjust your position to allow you to use your body weight to achieve the stretch. Now move yourself all the way down to the feet.

2

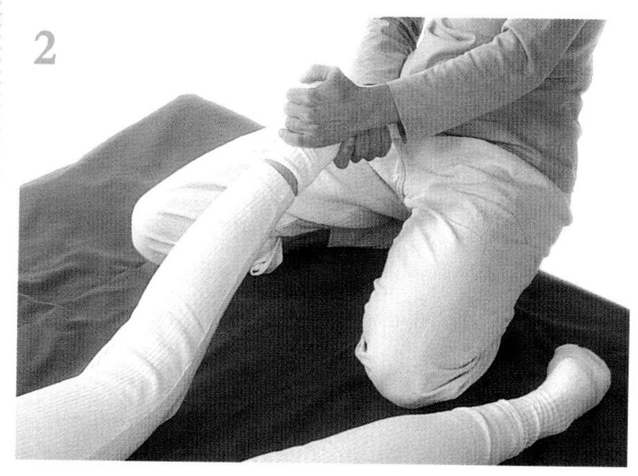

▲ With both hands, take a firm hold of the ankle, lean back and stretch out the leg to its full length.

Pressing the Sole

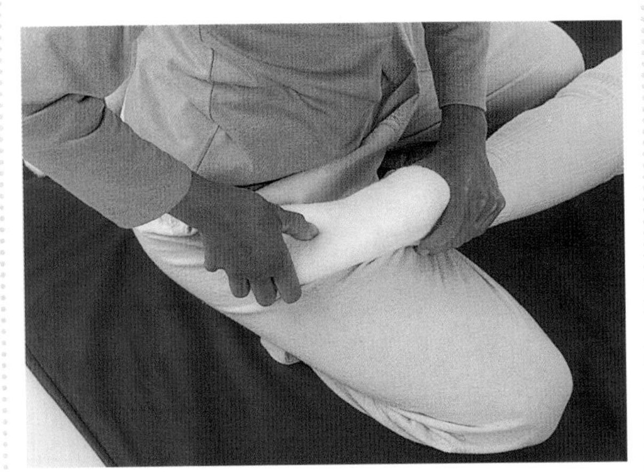

▲ Place your partner's foot in your lap and using your thumb apply pressure to KID 1 "Gushing Spring", one-third of the distance from the base of the second toe to the base of the heel.

Crossed Legs Stretch

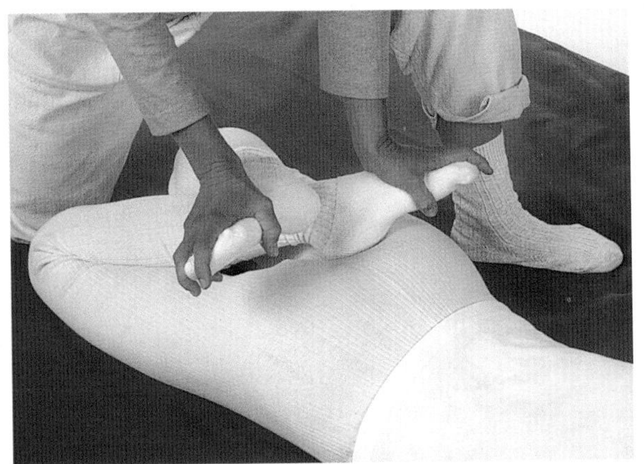

▲ Cross your partner's ankles and bring them slowly towards the buttocks. Do this stretch twice, the first time placing the more flexible leg in front (nearest to the buttocks) and then reversing this position for the second stretch. This also facilitates a smooth transition to the other side of your partner's body. Without losing contact with your partner, move over to the other leg and work through in the same way.

Walking on the Soles

▶ Stand up and walk on the soles of your partner's feet using your heels. Have the feet turned inwards and apply pressure to the soles with no weight on the toes. To complete the treatment, return to the starting position with your hand on your partner's sacrum. Reconnect to this area and then slowly break the contact with your partner.

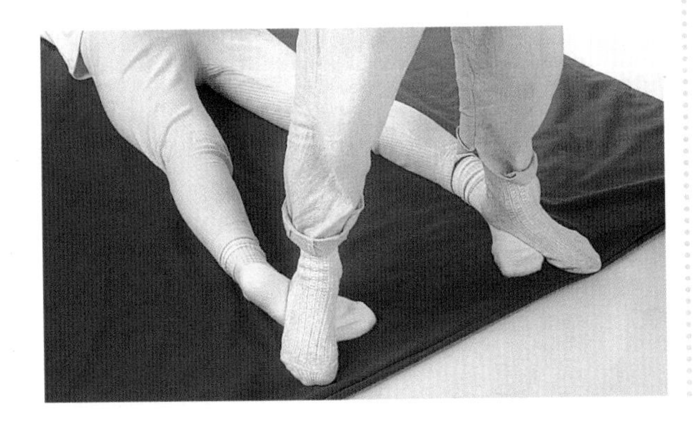

Respiratory System Enhancers: Self Help

The Lung energy controls our intake of fresh air and Ki from the external environment. During times of stress the bronchial tubes expand to let in more air and we tend to "over-breathe", or hyperventilate. Work on the Lung meridian and practise breathing exercises to enhance deeper breathing and a proper exchange of air with the environment.

These exercises will open up the chest and encourage an upright posture. You will feel your chest expanding and your breathing getting deeper as you practise the different movements. Try to breathe in through your nose and out through your mouth throughout the exercises.

Lung Stretch

▶ Link your index finger and thumb on both hands. Step forward with your right foot as you reach up towards the ceiling with your arms, opening them out to the sides slightly. Look up to the ceiling as you breathe in and feel the chest expanding as your lungs fill with air. Step back with your foot and relax your arms by your sides as you breathe out. Step forward again, this time with your left foot, and repeat the same movement. Repeat another three to four times on each side.

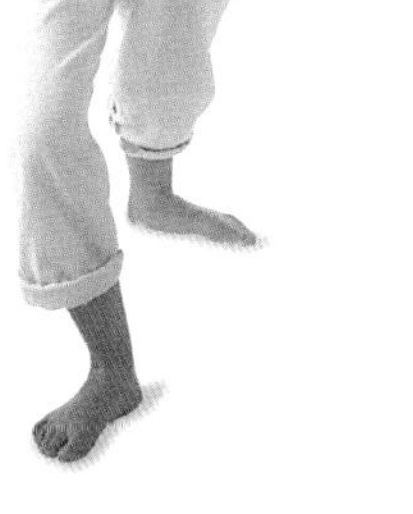

Chest Opening Exercise

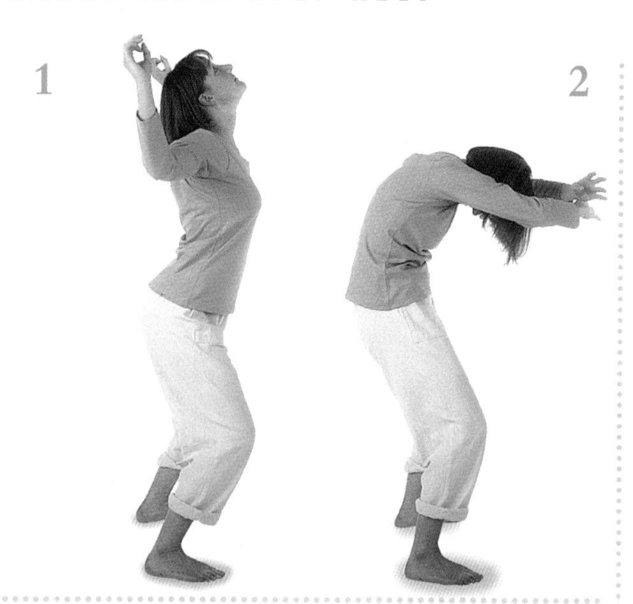

▶ Stand with your feet shoulder-width apart and knees bent. Lift your arms out to the sides with your elbows bent, and make loose fists with your hands. Take a deep breath in, opening your chest by bringing your arms back as much as possible.

▶ On the exhalation, cross your arms over in front of you and relax your head downwards. Keeping your knees bent, press the area in between your shoulder-blades backwards and feel the muscles stretching. Empty your breath out completely. Repeat the exercise four or five times.

Stretching the Lung and Large Intestine Meridians

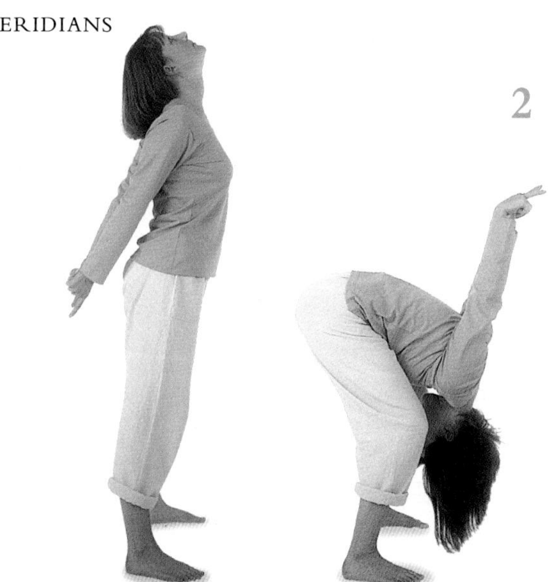

▶ Stand with your feet shoulder-width apart and knees bent and spread your feet slightly apart so that your toes are pointed outwards naturally. Hook your thumbs together behind your back, pointing the index fingers down to the floor. Inhale as you lift your head and look up towards the ceiling.

▶ On the exhalation, bend forward and stretch your arms back over your head, keeping the elbows straight. Bend down to a position that feels comfortable for you, without overstretching. Take a deep breath in and feel the stretch like a pulling sensation along the back of your legs, back and arms. Slowly exhale and relax. Stay down and repeat twice more, then slowly roll back up to standing and relax your arms.

Relaxation Position for Opening the Chest

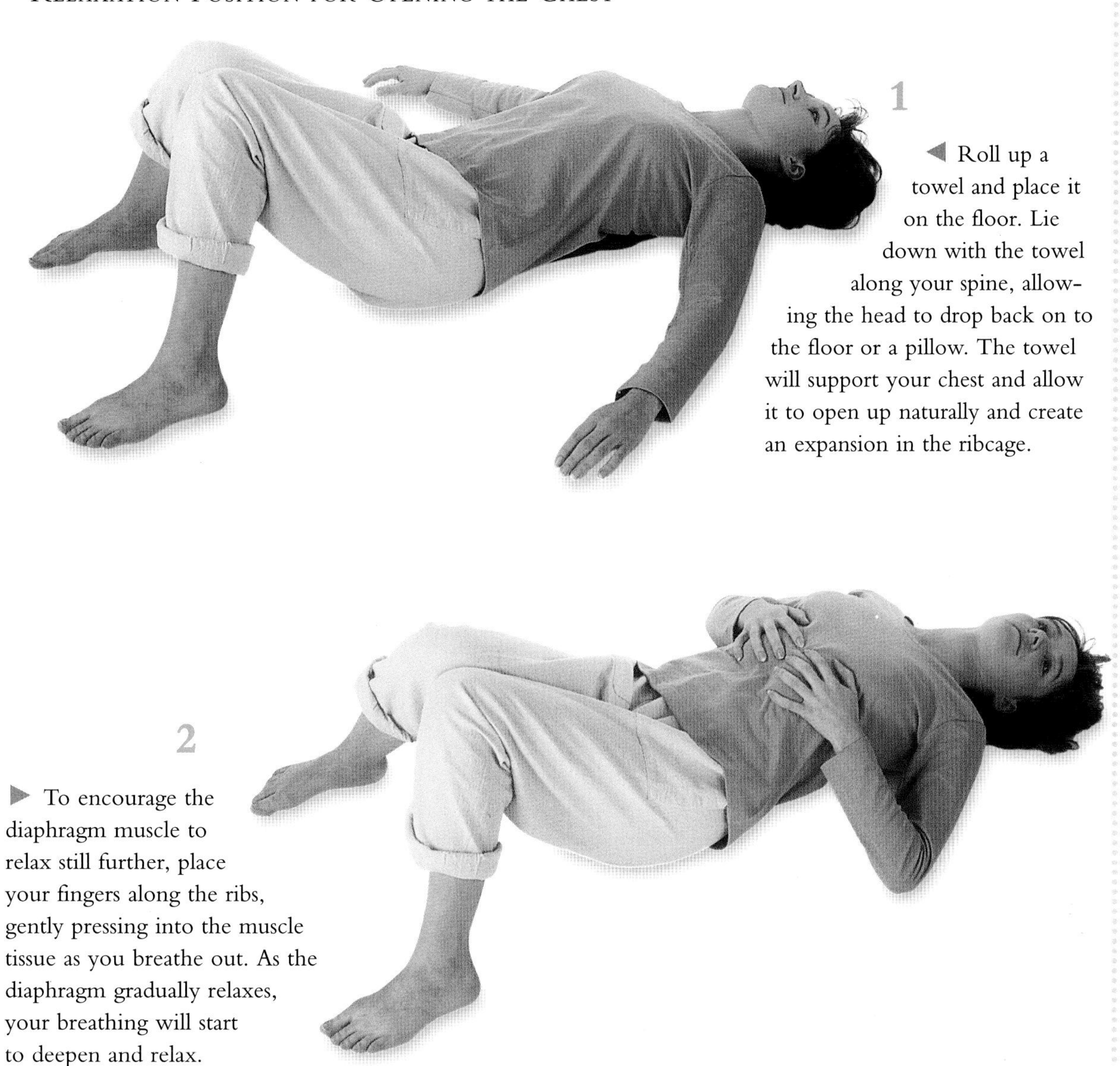

1

◀ Roll up a towel and place it on the floor. Lie down with the towel along your spine, allowing the head to drop back on to the floor or a pillow. The towel will support your chest and allow it to open up naturally and create an expansion in the ribcage.

2

▶ To encourage the diaphragm muscle to relax still further, place your fingers along the ribs, gently pressing into the muscle tissue as you breathe out. As the diaphragm gradually relaxes, your breathing will start to deepen and relax.

Respiratory System Enhancers: Improving Your Partner's Lung Energy

If your partner is feeling tired and stressed, experiencing tension in the upper body or suffers from shallow, rapid breathing, the following treatment will be very beneficial. It will help relaxation and promote deeper breathing, enchancing a better energy distribution to all parts of the body. Before proceeding with the treatment, place your hand on your partner's belly and give yourself time to tune into your partner's energy and breathing pattern. This area is thought of as the vital centre of the body and is called the *Hara*.

Diaphragm Release

▶ Place one hand underneath your partner's back in the area opposite the solar plexus and the other hand on top covering the area just below the sternum (breastbone). Focus into the area between your hands and encourage your partner to do the same. Feel the Ki from the breath of your partner reach this space, slowly allowing it to open and expand. You will gradually feel the tension go and the muscles relax to allow a deeper and more relaxed breathing.

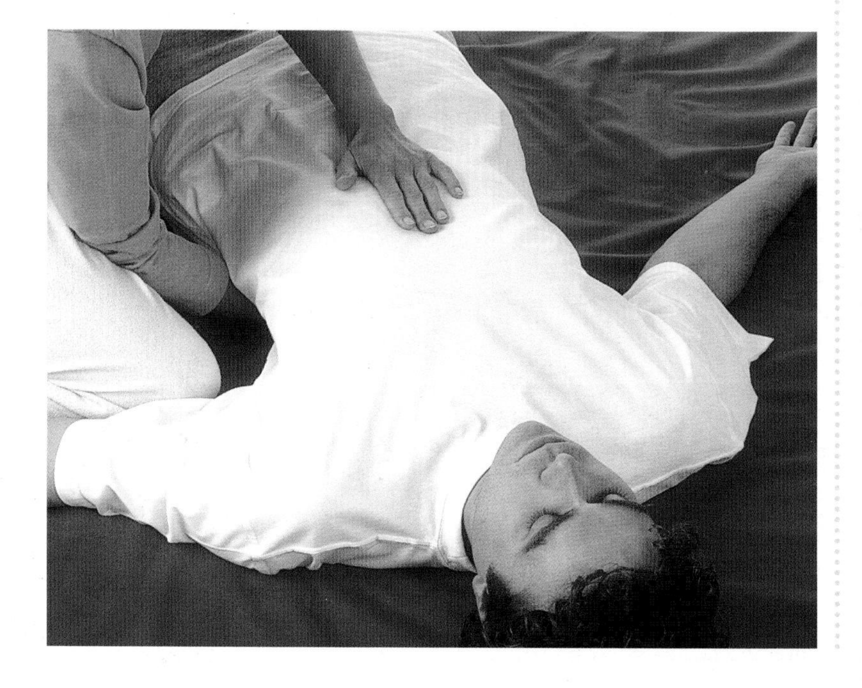

Opening Up the Chest

▶ Cross your arms over and place the palms of your hands on your partner's shoulders. Ask your partner to breathe in and on the out-breath bring your body weight over your hands, stimulating the first point of the Lung meridian and gently opening the chest. Repeat three times.

1

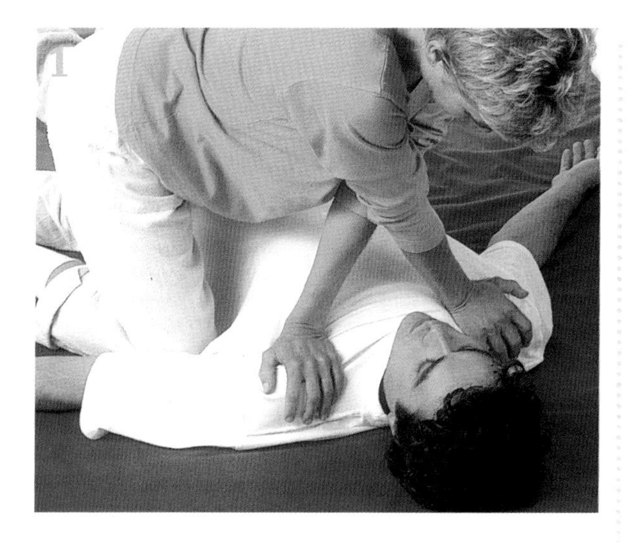

2

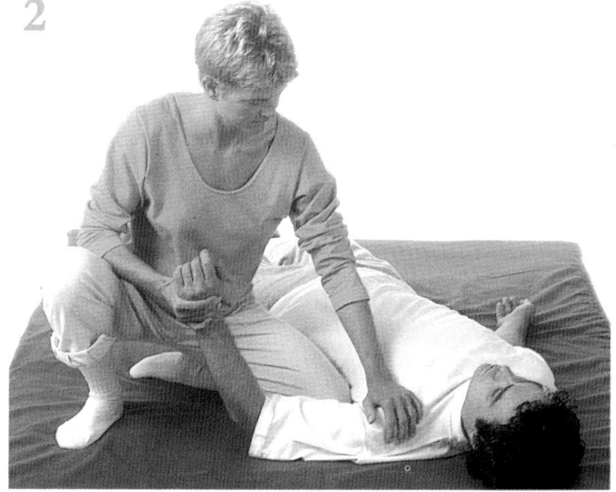

▲ Keep your left hand on the shoulder and take a firm hold of your partner's hand with your right hand. Lift the arm from the floor, shake it out and allow it to relax again.

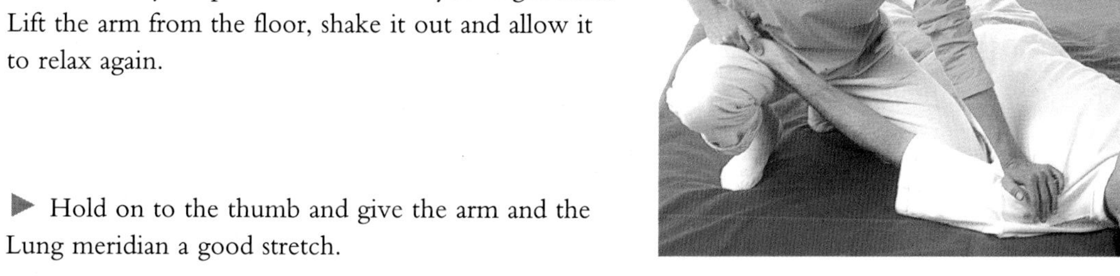

▶ Hold on to the thumb and give the arm and the Lung meridian a good stretch.

3

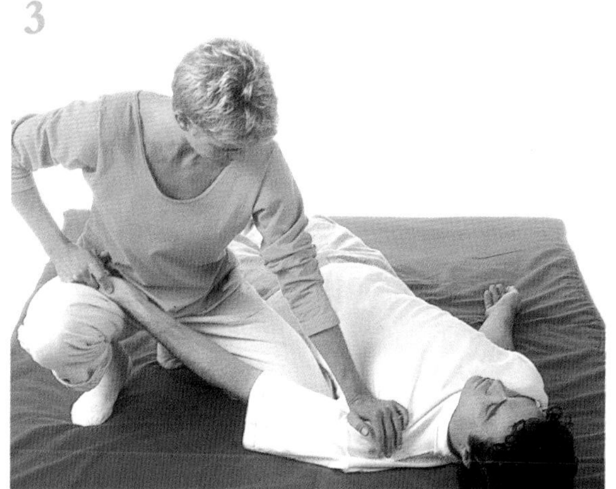

Palming Down the Lung Meridian

▶ Place your partner's arm at a 45-degree angle to the body. Use one of your hands to support the shoulder while the other hand palms along the arm to the hand. Stay on the thumb side of the arm to activate the energy in the Lung meridian.

1

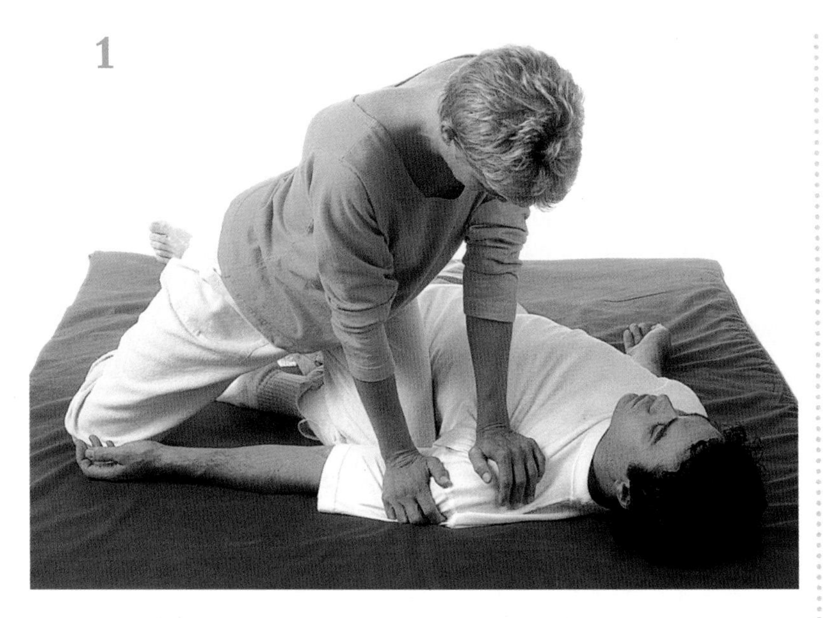

2

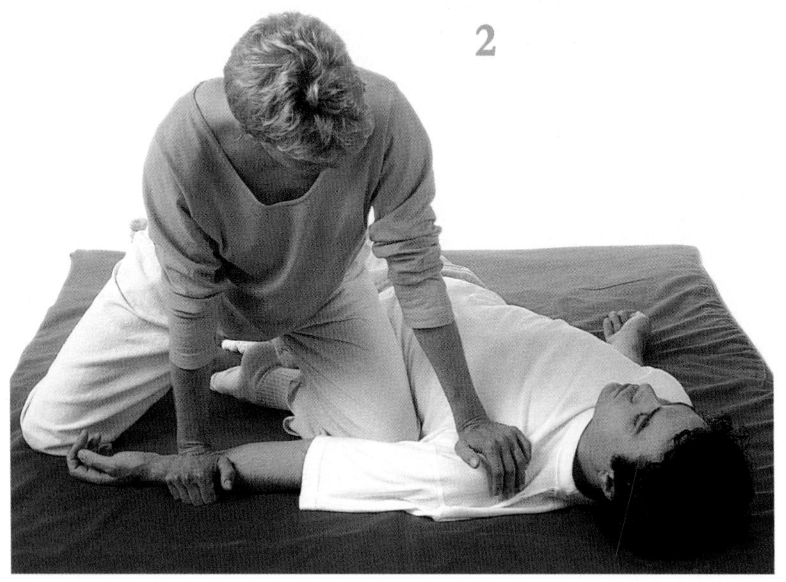

◀ Continue all the way down to the thumb (end point of the Lung channel). Avoid applying direct heavy pressure over the elbow joint.

Hand Treatment

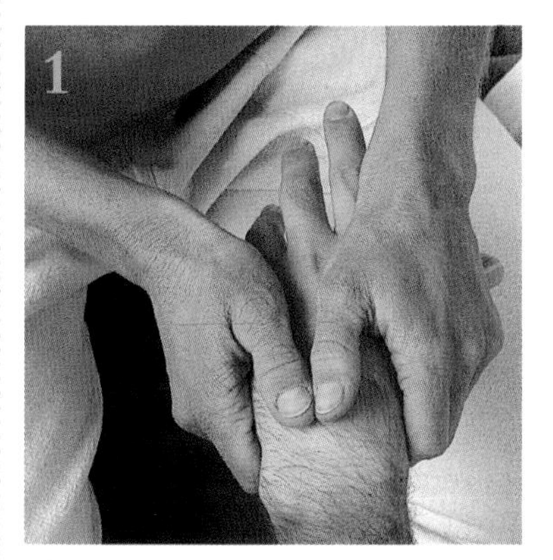

▲ Using your thumbs, massage the whole of the dorsal side of your partner's hand.

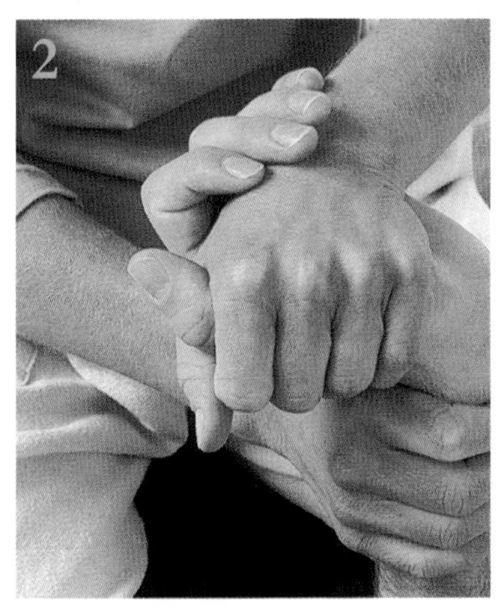

▲ Loosen up the wrist joint by rotating the hand.

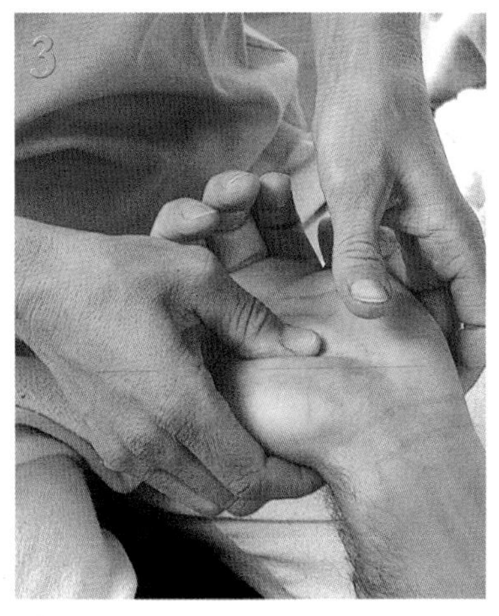

▲ Open up the palm of the hand and gently massage.

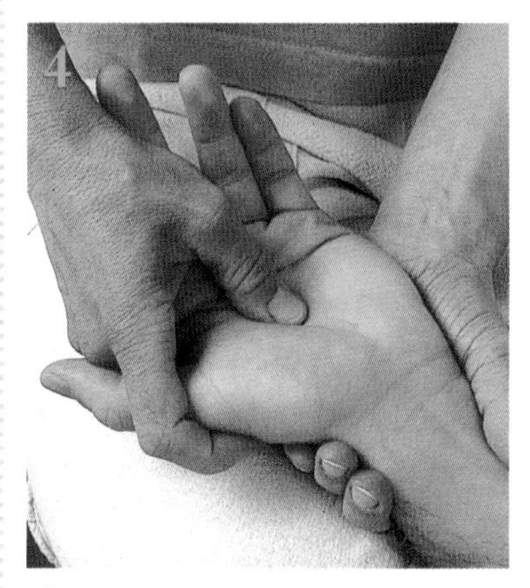

▲ Apply pressure to the point in the centre of the palm, called "Palace of Anxiety". A very good point for calming and releasing tension in hands and upper body.

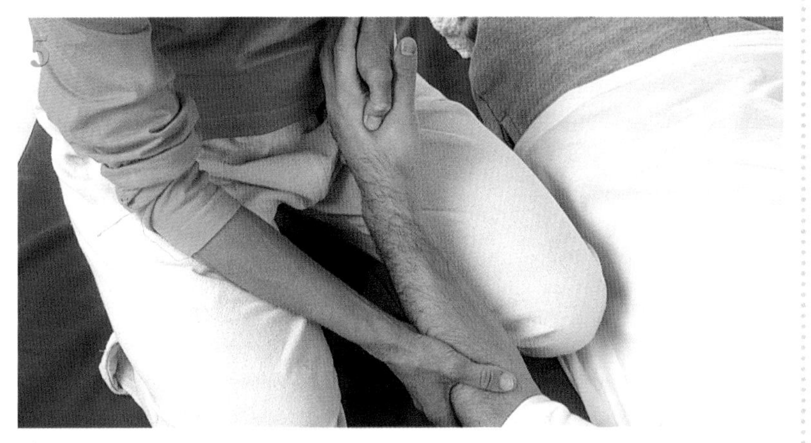

▲ Find point LI4 which is located in the web between the index finger and thumb. Stimulating this point with gentle thumb pressure will lift headaches and help clear any mucous congestion in the lungs.

Rotating the Arm

▶ Hold your partner's arm by the wrist and support the shoulder with your other hand. Step forward and rotate the arm into an overhead stretch. Before you step forward, you need to apply pressure into the supporting hand at the shoulder, maintaining this pressure to ensure a strong stretch. Step back, allowing the arm to return to the starting position. Repeat three times, shaking and loosening the shoulder between each stretch to relax it.

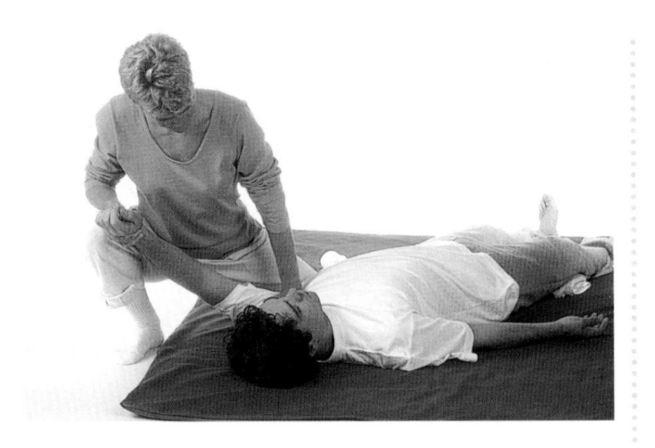

Overhead Stretch

1

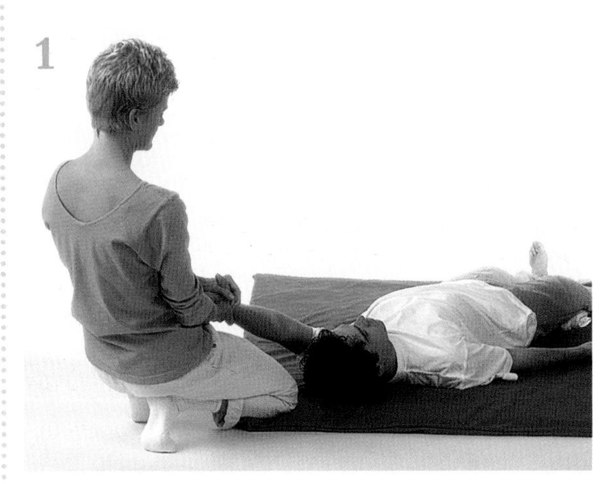

▲ Kneel behind your partner, facing your partner's head. Grip their hand and support the wrist to achieve a maximum stretch by leaning backwards, using your body weight. Reach down to take hold of your partner's other hand.

2

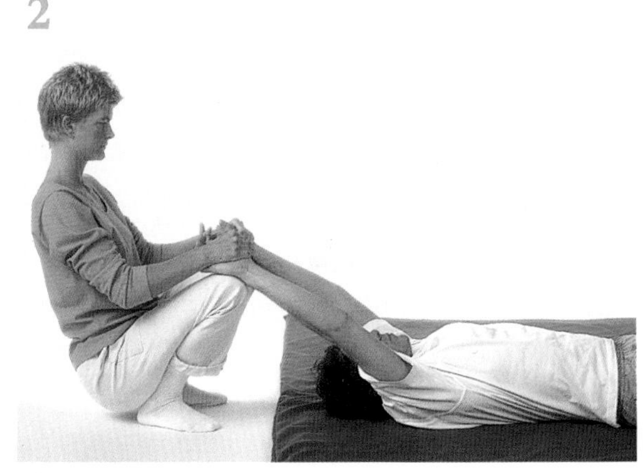

▲ Place both hands on top of your knees and stretch the arms by leaning backwards. Let go of the arm you have treated and move over to the other side. Repeat the whole sequence working on the other arm. To finish, reconnect with your partner's *Hara*.

Stretching the Lungs

These three stretches will open up the chest and shoulder girdle allowing for greater intake of air and Ki. Your partner will feel the expansion of the chest and the exercises will encourage deeper, more relaxed, breathing. Repeat each stretch three to four times.

► Stand behind your partner, sitting with legs stretched in front, the side of your leg against the spine. Take hold of the hands, gripping around the thumbs, and as you both exhale, lift up from your knees and lean backwards until your partner feels the stretch.

1

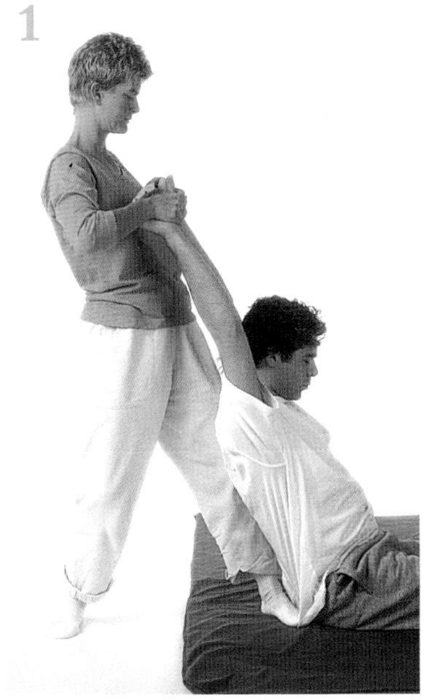

2

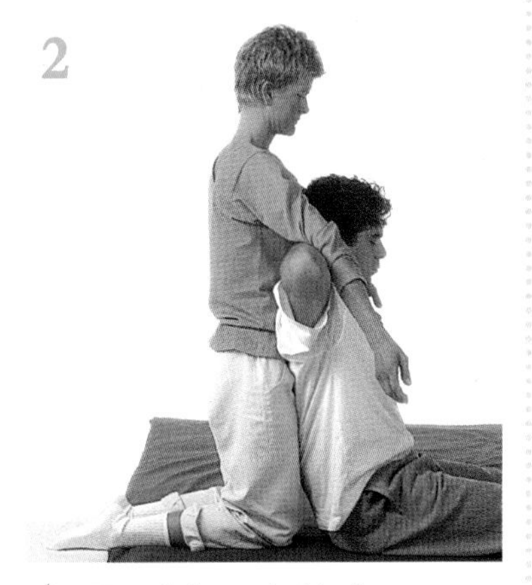

▲ Kneel down behind your partner and ask them to clasp the hands behind the neck. Bring your arms in front of your partner's arms, and on the out-breath gently open up the elbows to the sides, allowing your partner to feel the chest opening.

3

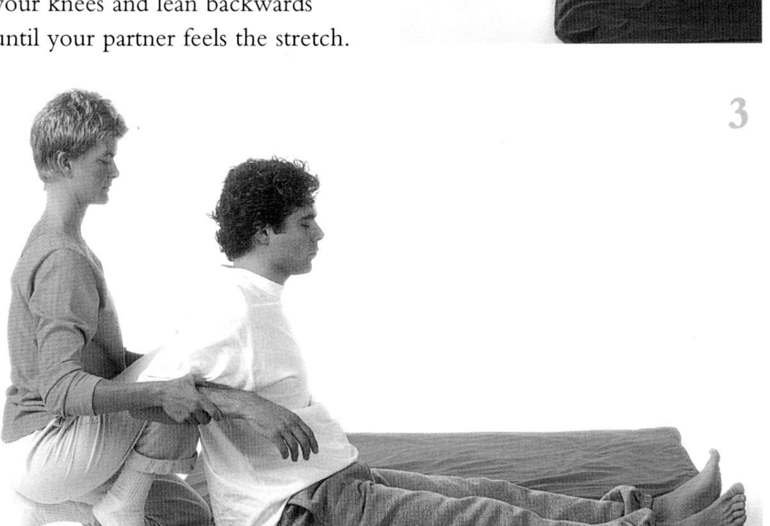

◄ Bring one knee up to support the lower back. Take hold of your partner's lower arms, and on the out-breath bring the elbows towards each other behind your partner's back.

Digestive Balancers: Self Help

Long-term effects of stress may be evident in your digestive system and peristalsis, leaving you with constipation, diarrhoea or abdominal cramps. To help and support your digestive system, you need to eat a well-balanced diet rich in fibres, grains and fresh vegetables. Chew your food well so that it is in a liquid form before it reaches your stomach, and try to drink between meals rather than with your food. Give yourself time for regular exercise, and practise the following Ampuku massage exercises to stimulate the digestive process.

Self Ampuku

This routine will gently massage your large intestine and give some support to the peristaltic movements of your bowels.

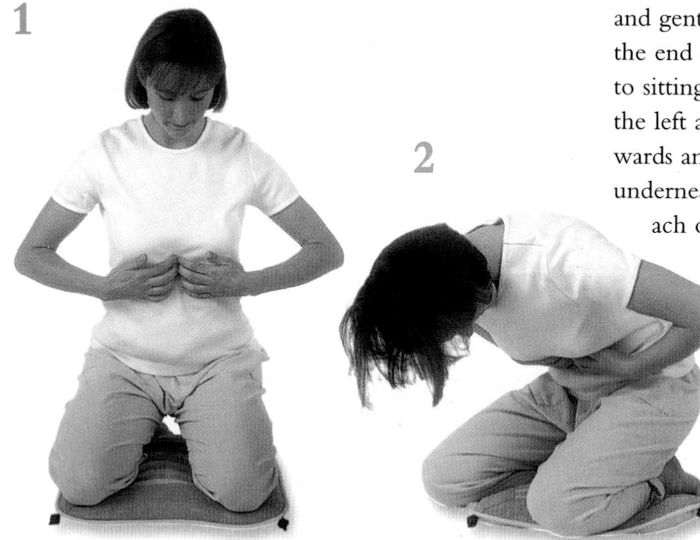

◀ Sit on a chair or kneel on a cushion on the floor. Apply your fingers to the area just below your solar plexus. Spread your fingers out under the ribcage and take a deep breath in.

▼ On the out-breath, lean forward from the waist and gently press your fingers up and under the ribs. At the end of the exhalation, relax completely and roll up to sitting position again. Move your hands slightly to the left and repeat the same breathing, leaning forwards and working with your fingers into the area underneath the left side of your ribs where your stomach organ is. Exhale completely, relax and roll up to sitting again. Move your hands further down on the left-hand side of your abdomen, to the area between your ribs and your hip bone. Repeat the same technique here, then move to the area inside your left hip bone and do the same thing. Continue all the way around your abdomen in a clockwise direction until you come back to the starting point.

Working on the Digestive System

The Stomach and Spleen energy channels are associated with functions of ingestion and digestion of food and information for mental and physical nourishment. In traditional Chinese medicine, the Stomach corresponds to the entire digestive tract, from the mouth to the small intestine and is a vital Organ for the production of Ki energy in the body.

The following 20-minute Shiatsu routine is ideal for treating symptoms such as indigestion a bloated stomach and abdominal cramps or pain due to stress.

Tuning In

▶ Sit in the Seiza position at your partner's side and gently place your right hand on the lower *Hara* and your left hand on the side. Take a few moments of stillness to "tune in" and observe. Be aware of any tension and note the breathing rate: fast and shallow indicates tension; slow and deep shows relaxation.

Trace the borderlines of your partner's *Hara*. Start at the ribcage just below the breastbone and move out to the sides and then to the pelvic region.

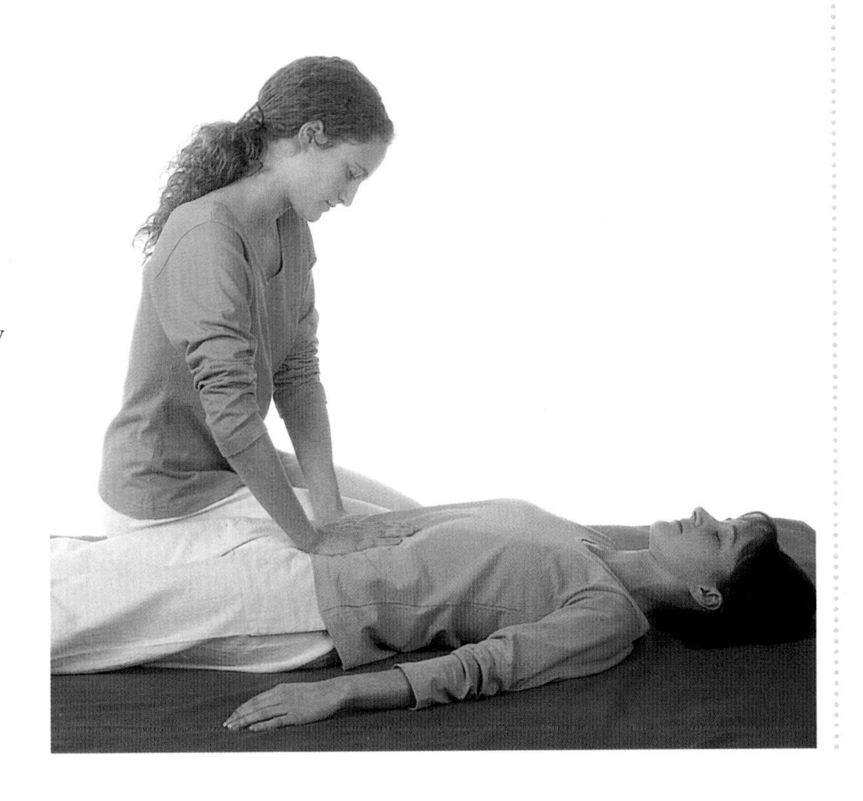

Ampuku Abdominal Massage

These techniques will stimulate the movements of the large intestine and are good to use for relieving constipation and stomach pain.

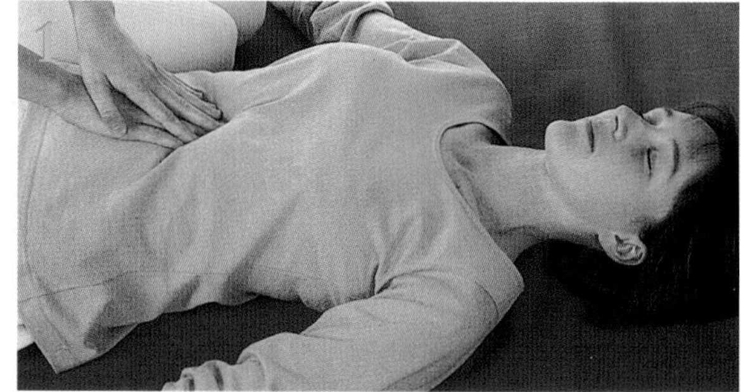

▲ Using two hands, one on top of the other, apply finger-pad pressure in a clockwise movement around the *Hara*. Where you find tension, apply gradually deeper pressure to dissolve the tension.

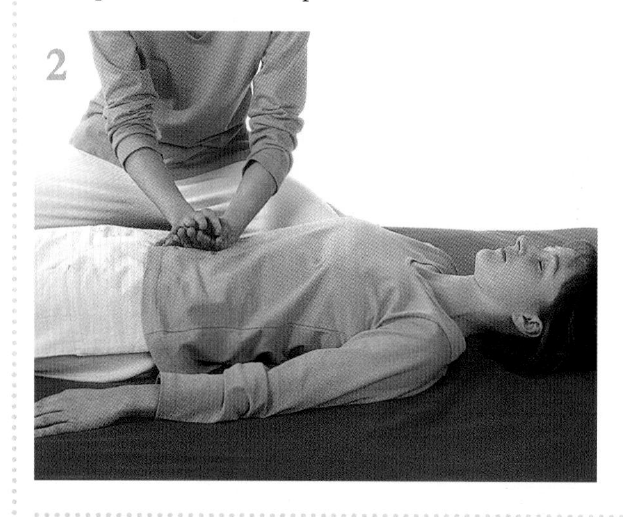

◀ With one hand on top of the other, make a rocking and pushing type motion like rolling dough, from one side of the *Hara* to the other and pull back using the heel of the hand. Repeat until the *Hara* relaxes.

Rotating the Hip Joint

▶ Keep one hand on the *Hara* while the other holds the right leg just below the knee.

▶ Move from your centre, using your whole body, not just your arm muscles, to rotate your partner's leg. Keep a fixed distance between your chest and your partner's knee to ensure a balanced rotation of the hip. This will loosen up the hip joint.

1

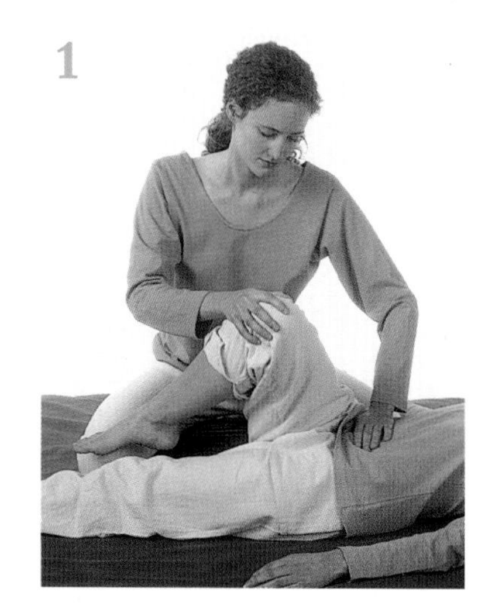

2

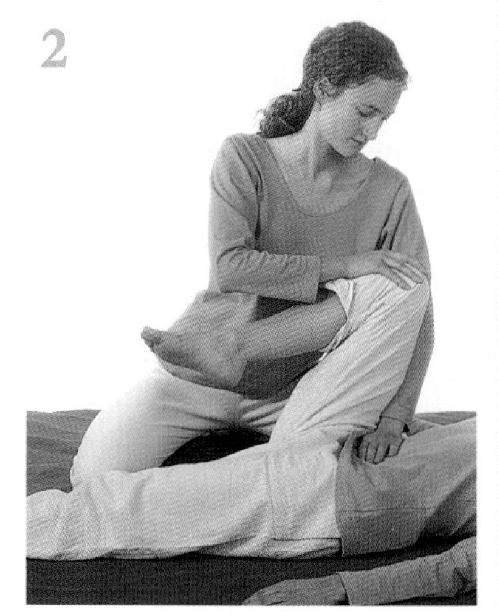

Palming

▼ Stretch your partner's leg out, and place your knee underneath your partner's knee for support or use a pillow. Apply palm pressure along the outside frontal edge of the leg following the Stomach meridian. Start from the top of the thigh and work down to the foot. Repeat three times.

1

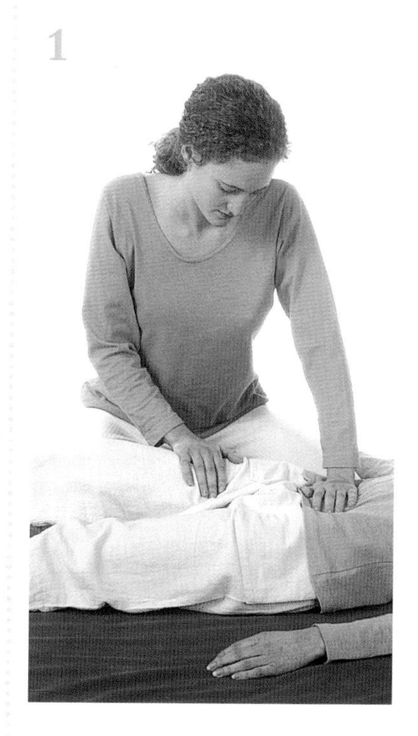

2

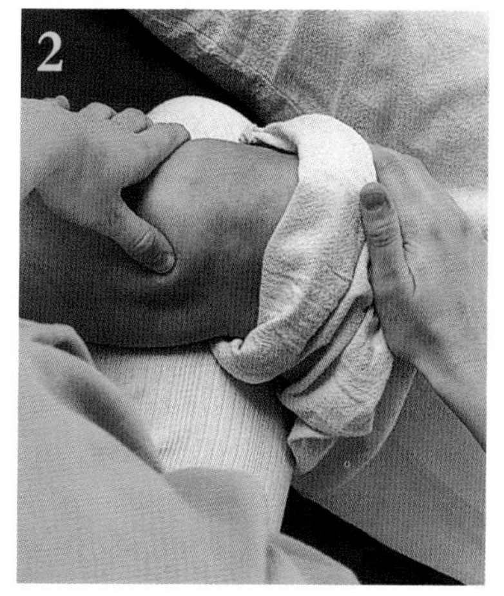

▲ Stimulate ST36, "Leg Three Miles", using thumb pressure. The point is located four fingers' width below the knee-cap on the outside of the shin-bone. The name refers to this point's remarkable effect: it has been used since ancient times to build up strength and endurance.

Stretching the Leg

▼ Move down to your partner's feet and take a firm hold of the right ankle. Stretch the leg out by leaning back. Make contact with both feet and move to the left leg. Bend the leg and start rotating the hip joint. Repeat the whole sequence treating the left leg.

To complete the treatment come back to the *Hara*. Tune in again and check for tension/relaxation in the *Hara* as well as in the breathing. Has it changed?

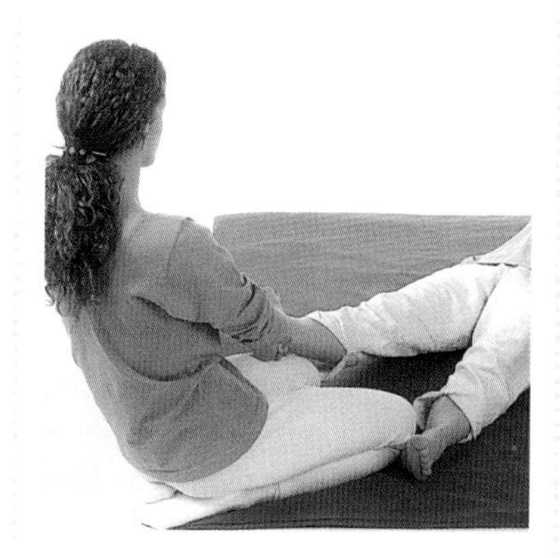

Lymph and Immune System Revivers: With a Partner

The immune system includes your spleen, thymus gland and lymph nodes. It is responsible for moving proteins and fats around the body. It is also responsible for filtering body fluids, producing white blood cells and immunity. If you are subject to stress over a long period of time, it will weaken your immune system, leaving you vulnerable to viral infections. According to Oriental medicine, the Spleen function of transforming and transporting energy is the main influence on your lymphatic system. These simple Shiatsu techniques will help to awaken your immune and lymphatic systems.

Lymphatic Pump

► This technique will enhance the removal of toxic waste substances from the body and will improve the circulation of antibodies. Ask your partner to lie down on the back with legs straight. Place your palms over the soles of your partner's feet. Intermittently rock the feet towards the head in a rhythmic motion of about two movements per second for 3-4 minutes. This relaxes your partner and assists the movement of lymphatic fluid through the body.

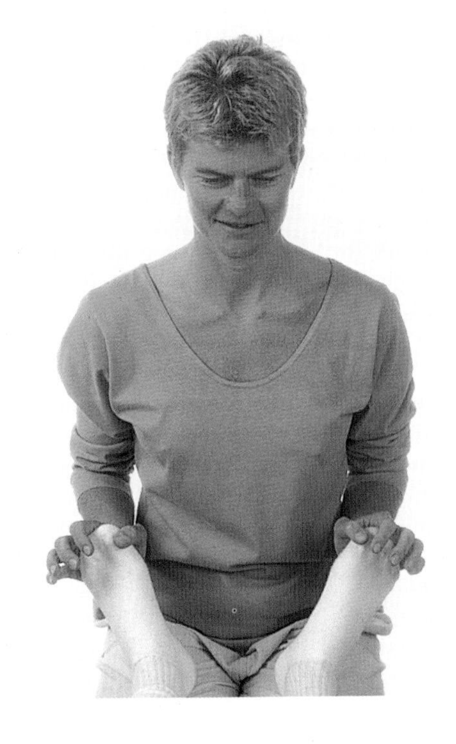

Rotating the Hip Joint

▶ Bend your partner's leg and move yourself up to the side. Bring one hand to the *Hara* and hold the leg just below the knee with the other hand. Slowly rotate the hip joint, moving from the centre of yourself. Keep a fixed distance between your chest and your partner's knee to ensure a balanced rotation of the hip.

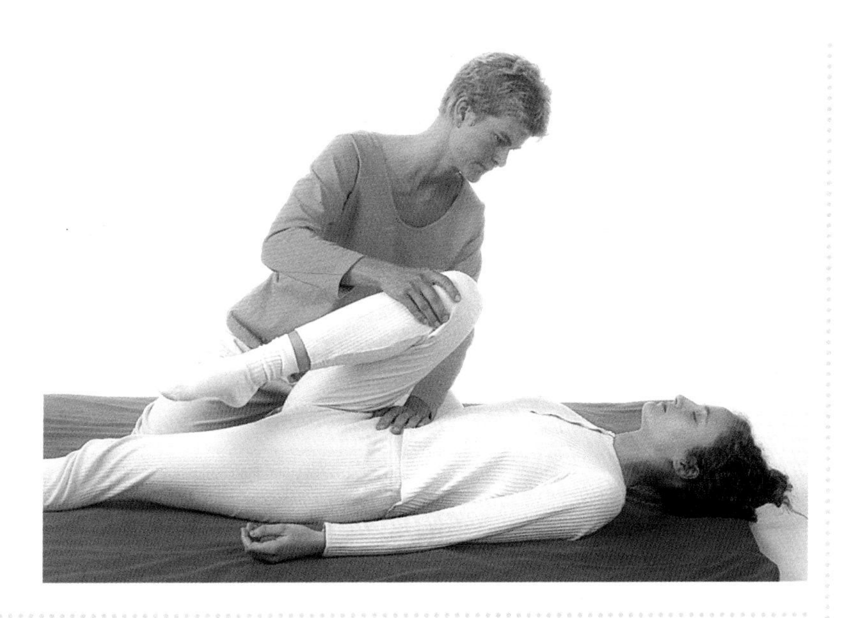

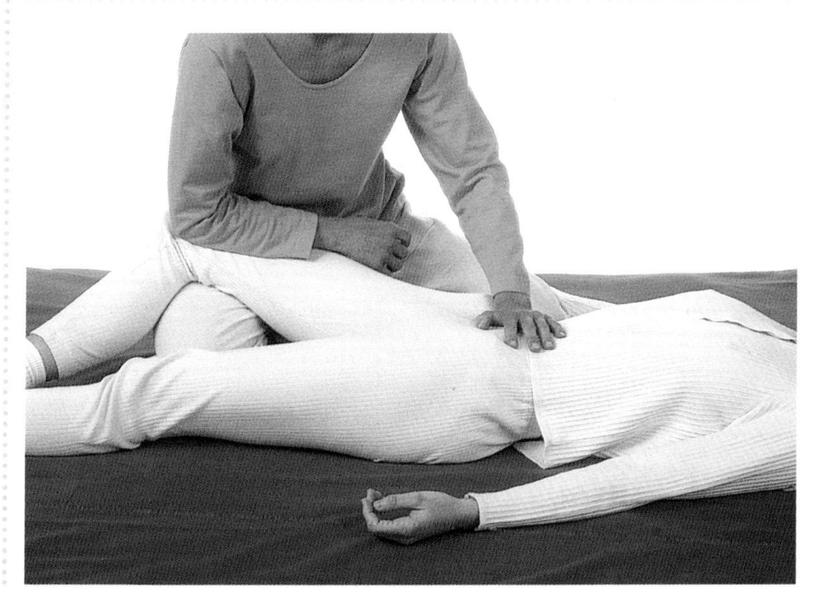

Opening the Spleen Meridian

◀ Place your partner's foot against the opposite inside ankle so that the leg is bent, exposing the inside leg. Use a pillow or your own knee to support the leg to avoid groin strain. Keeping one hand on the *Hara*, ask your partner to inhale and gently use your forearm to stretch open the Spleen meridian on the out-breath.

Treating the Spleen Meridian

▶ Support the lower leg with a cushion and, starting from the inside of your partner's big toe, use your thumb to apply perpendicular pressure along the medial part of the foot.

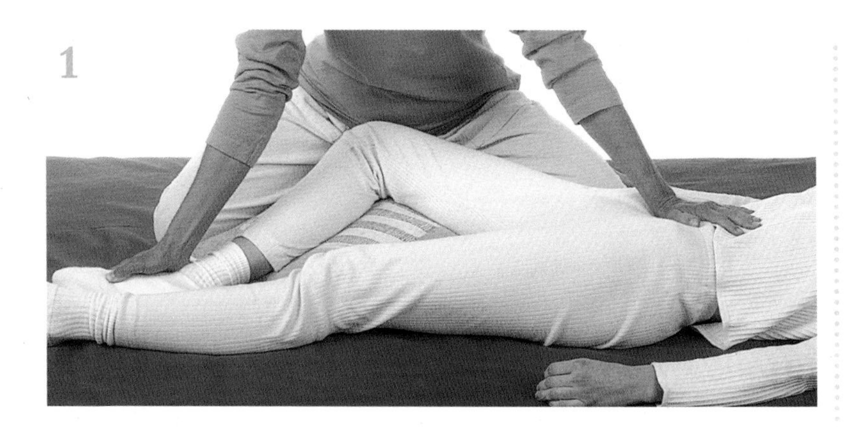

1

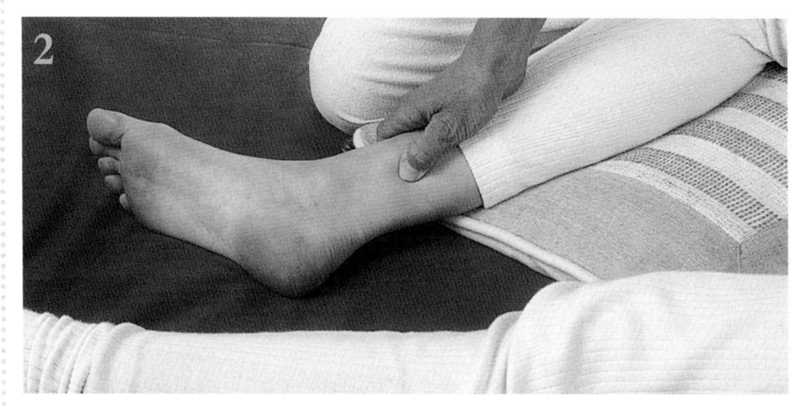

2

◀ Four fingers' width above the medial ankle bone on the inside of the shin bone is SP6, "Three Yin Junction". The name refers to this point's intersection with the three Yin channels of the foot. Press this point to regulate the energy in the Spleen channel and help treat insomnia, digestive problems and menstrual disorders.

▶ At the top of the shin bone on the medial side of the leg is SP9, another powerful point on the Spleen meridian. Press this point to treat abdominal and menstrual pain, or local pain in the knee.

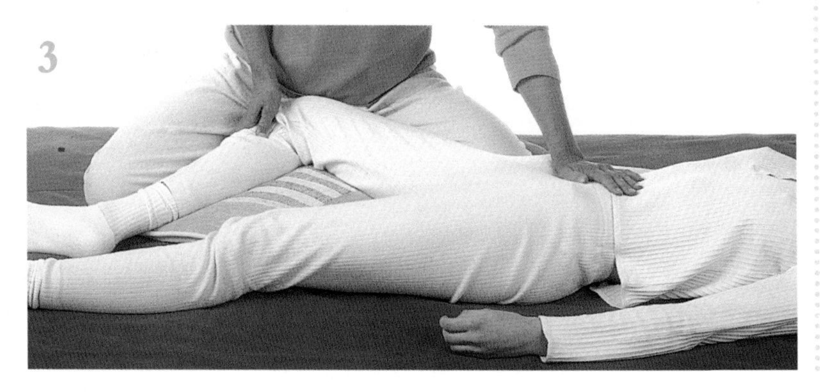

3

4

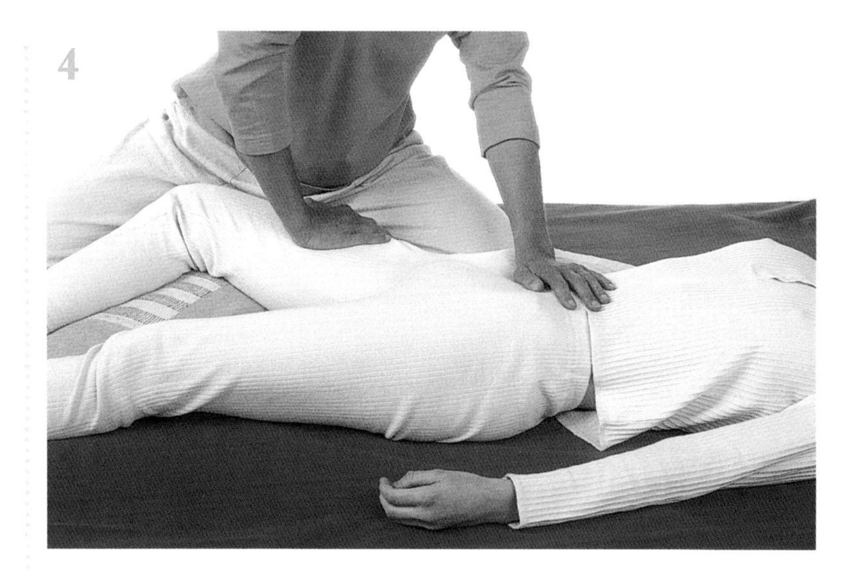

◀ Continue to treat the Spleen meridian in the thigh. Use a gentle pressure and treat all the way to the groin using the heel of the hand.

Double Leg Rotation

▶ Rotate one leg and then bend the other leg as well. Come to a standing position, bring your feet close to your partner's hips for support and gently bring the knees to the chest. Ease up on the stretch and rotate both legs. Move over to the other side, stretch out your partner's right leg on the floor and repeat the same routine on the left side.

To complete your treatment of the Lymph and Immune System, come back to your partner's *Hara*.

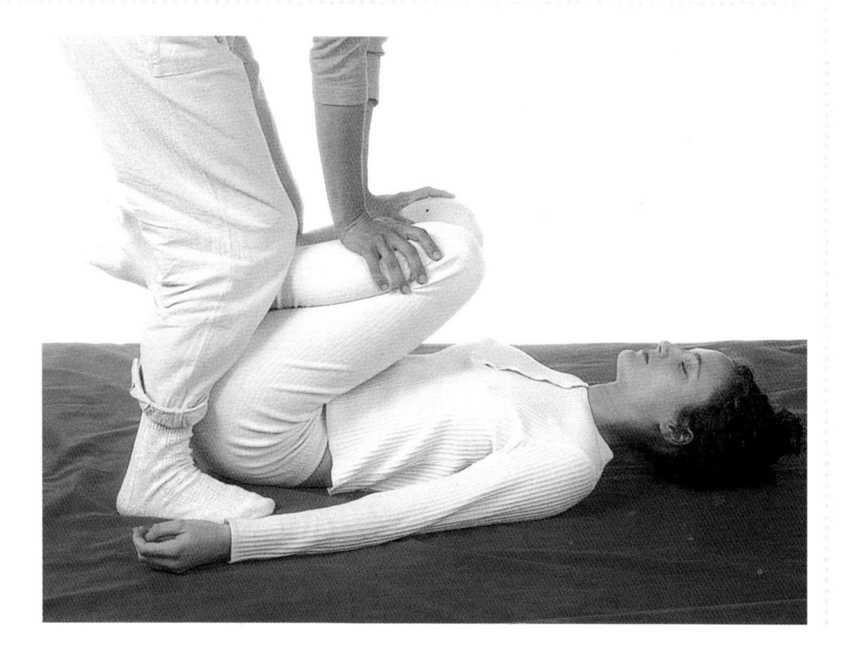

CIRCULATORY SYSTEM ENHANCERS

The Heart organ and the Heart and Heart Governor channels are the central focuses for regulating circulation and maintenance of the blood, according to traditional Chinese medicine. The condition of the Heart Ki is weakened by poor diet, lack of exercise and excessive heat.

The internal heat of passion can also injure the Heart energy. In extreme cases, repressed emotion gradually builds up in the body and rises to the chest as a heart attack.

Disturbed Heart energy may lead to conditions like poor sleep pattern, disturbed concentration, anxiety, hypertension and nervous stress. Shiatsu will help calm the mind and prevent these problems.

TREATING THE HEART MERIDIAN

▶ The Heart meridian is located on the inside of the arm and can be treated in the same way as you treat the Lung meridian (see under Respiratory system), with the arm in a slightly different position. The Heart meridian starts in the axilla (armpit) and runs along the ulnar (little finger) side of the arm to the little finger. To expose the energy channel, place your partner's arm with the hand above the head, palm facing upwards. Support the elbow with a cushion, kneel in an open Seiza position and work from the *Hara* in your movements.

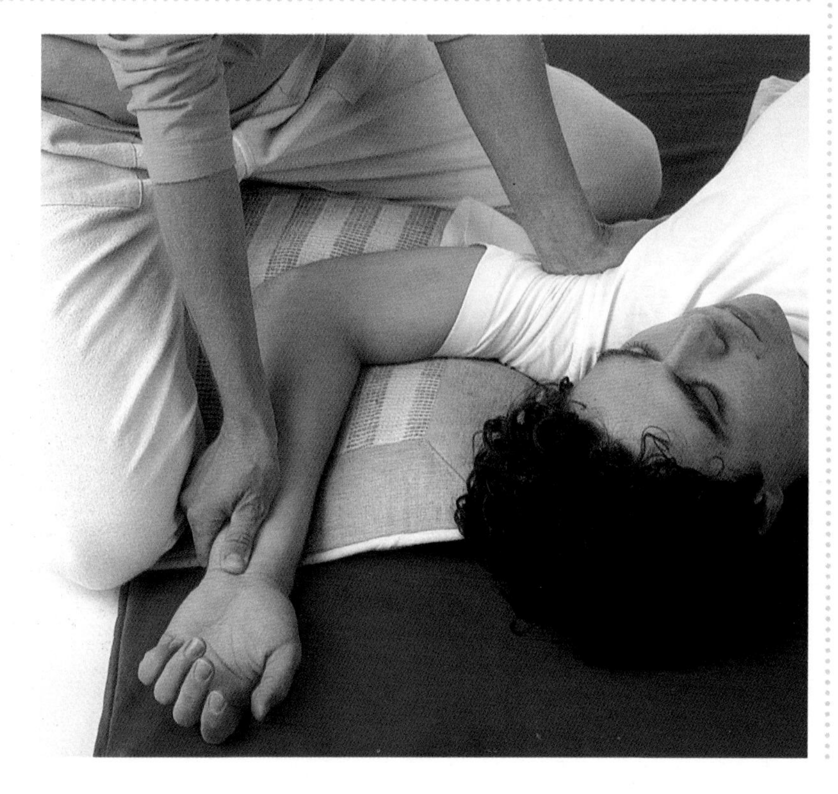

Heart Stretch

To stretch out and balance the energy in the Heart meridian, practise the following exercise.

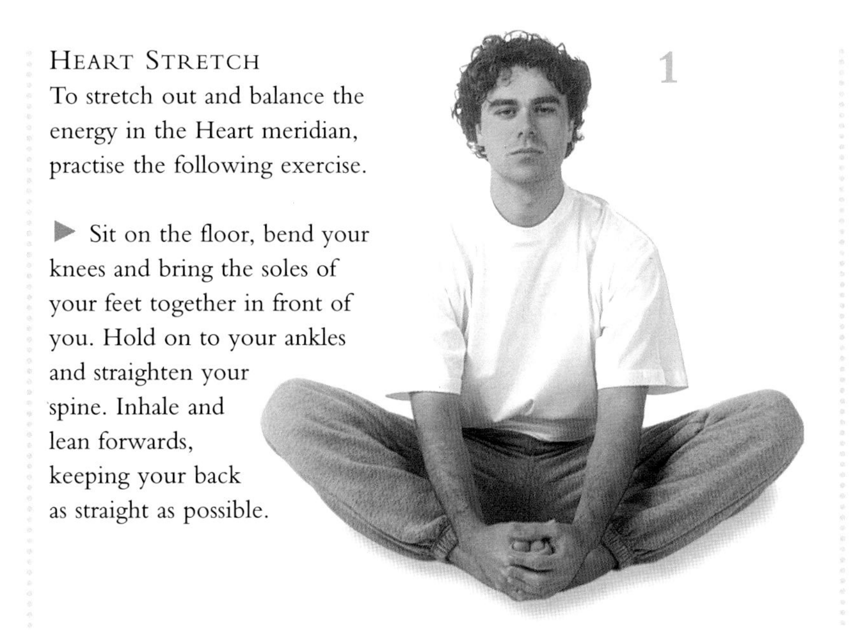

1

▶ Sit on the floor, bend your knees and bring the soles of your feet together in front of you. Hold on to your ankles and straighten your spine. Inhale and lean forwards, keeping your back as straight as possible.

▶ Breathe out as you bring your head towards your feet and your elbows in front of your legs. Open up the axilla (armpit) and relax into the position. Take another three deep breaths in and out in this position, then roll back up to sitting again.

2

Body Scrub

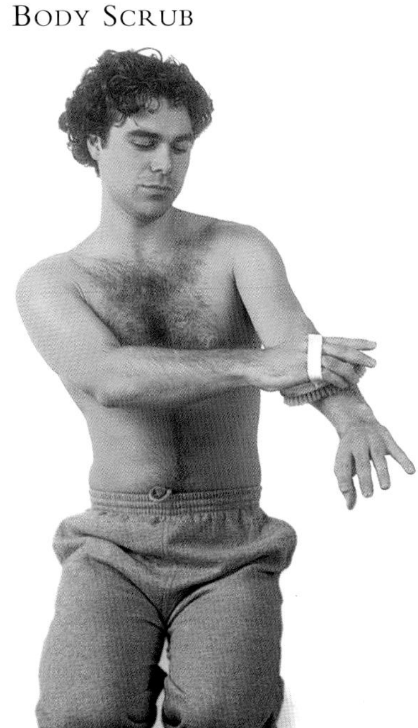

▲ To improve the blood circulation to the skin generally and to the peripheries in particular, give yourself a daily body scrub. Use a dry loofah, skin brush, rough face flannel or towel. Cover your whole body, rubbing your skin vigorously until the area becomes reddened, as blood comes to the surface. This technique will also assist in the elimination of toxins and dead skin cells.

Kenbiki Techniques

These are basically skin pulling, squeezing, pinching and rubbing techniques that are very useful in activating better blood and Ki circulation to an area. They go deeper than simply rubbing over the skin surface, with the intention of stimulating and releasing tension in the tissue below the skin. Not only is circulation affected, activating the Heart Ki, but also the sensory nerves and the oil and sweat glands.

Kenbiki techniques are commonly applied to the back muscles, which tend to become restricted by tension. Since these muscles are responsible for holding you upright and balancing your body, restrictions cause postural imbalances which in turn may affect your organ functions, especially those of the pelvis. Pinching and squeezing the muscles along the spine is invigorating and relaxing and assists the trunk nerve communication to your organs.

Palm Rubbing

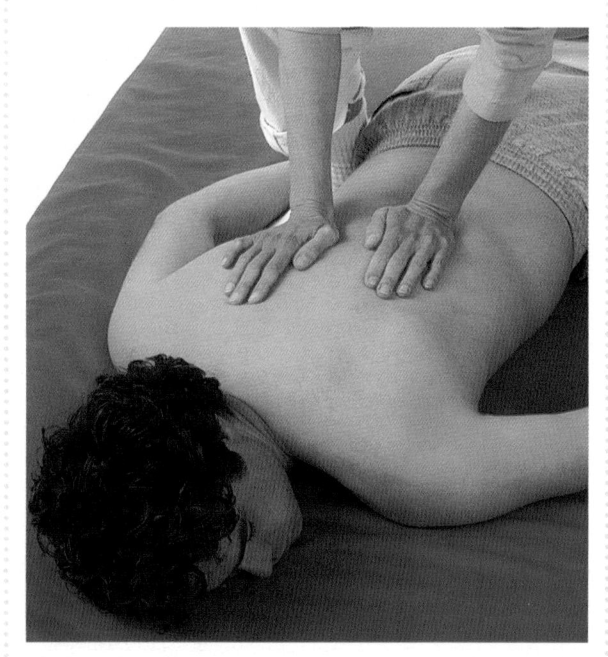

▲ Using both palms, apply pressure and rub down either side of the spine.

Rubbing

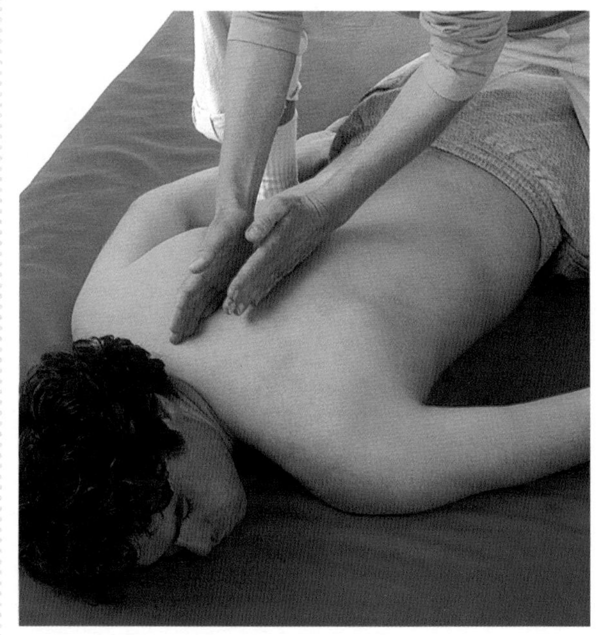

▲ Using the little finger side of your hands, vigorously rub down either side of the spine a few times until the area reddens.

Rolling the Skin

▼ Pinch and take hold of the skin on the lower part of the spine (lumbar area). Lift the tissue and gradually "roll" it up the spine. Repeat three or four times.

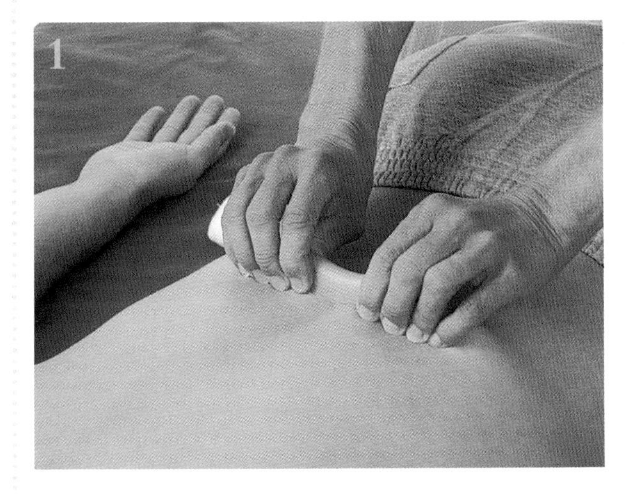

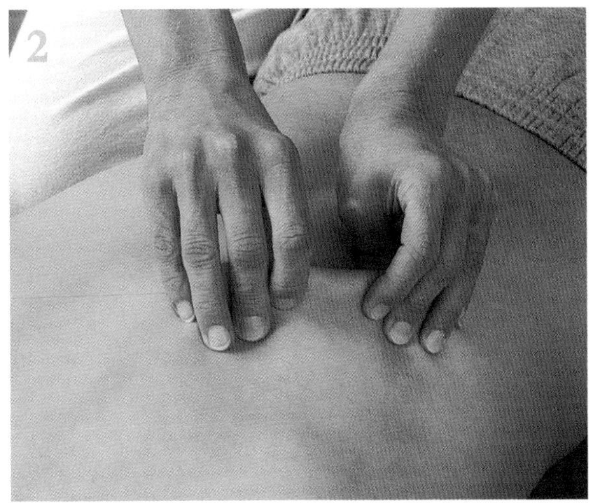

▲ "Roll" the skin from the spine, the centre line, out towards the sides to cover the entire back.

Pinching

▶ Use your index and middle fingers to pinch and take hold of the tissue. Twist and lift the skin at the same time. Work within your partner's pain threshold. Cover the whole back using this technique. You will see the area redden as the blood circulation improves, and your partner will have a sense of warmth spreading across their back.

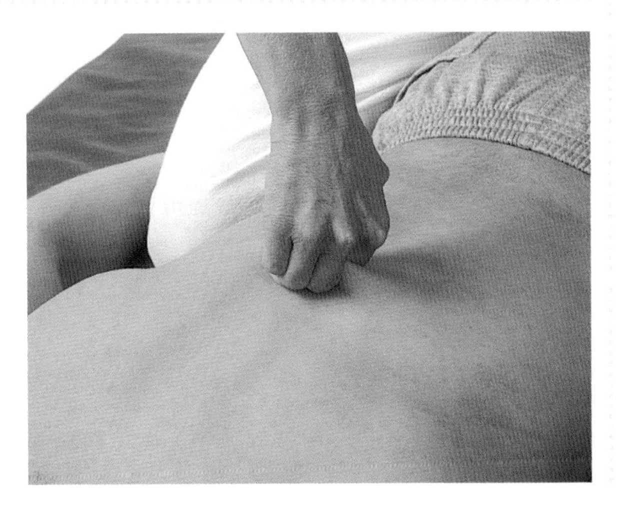

Tension Relievers

When you are under stress your centre of gravity tends to shift from the abdominal area up to the chest, causing tension in the neck and shoulders and often resulting in a feeling of a heaviness on your shoulders. Imagine how wonderful it would be to have someone touch these areas and relieve some of the pain and discomfort. To complete your Shiatsu session, pay some attention to these specific areas of your partner, or give your friend at work a neck and shoulder treatment there and then, in a chair.

Tuning In

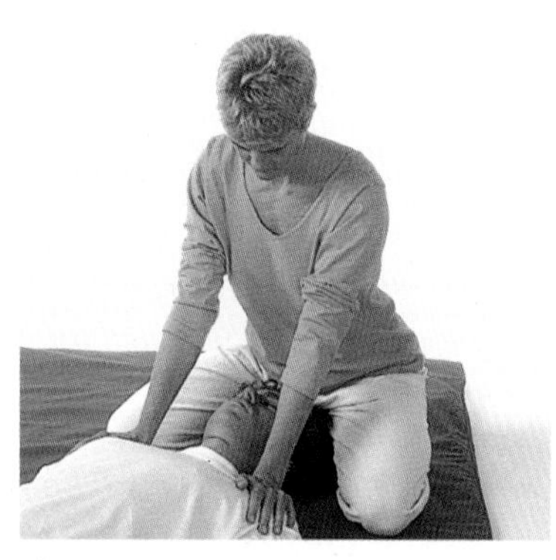

▲ Sit down in the Seiza position at your partner's head. Place your hands on the shoulders and tune in. Be aware of the breathing and state of relaxation before you start. Ask your partner to breathe in and on the exhalation apply a bit of pressure to the shoulders by leaning into your arms. Repeat a few times. This opens up the chest and encourages relaxation.

Kneading the Shoulders

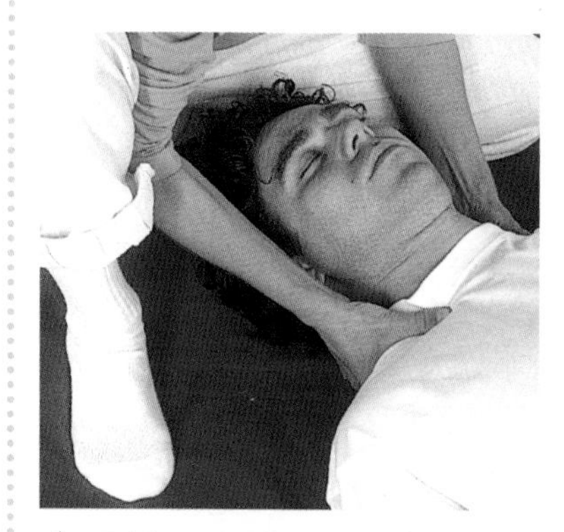

▲ With your fingers underneath and thumbs on top, gently and firmly massage the shoulders using a kneading action. Feel the tension in the muscles relaxing and the tissue gradually softening up.

Neck Stretch

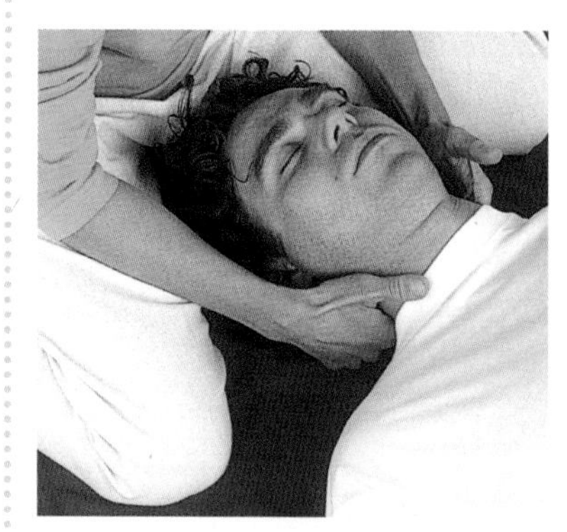

▲ Move your hands to the neck. With your thumbs on the side and fingers underneath, stretch out the neck by gently pulling away. Repeat a few times until you feel the neck muscles relax.

Squeezing the Neck

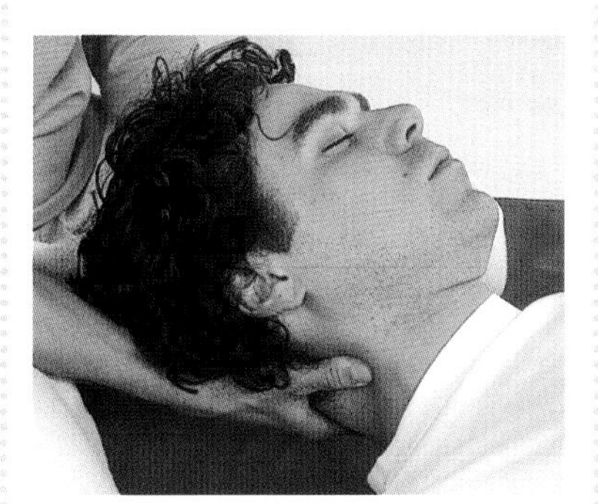

▲ Lift your partner's head off the floor and firmly squeeze the muscles of the neck.

Releasing Muscle Tendons

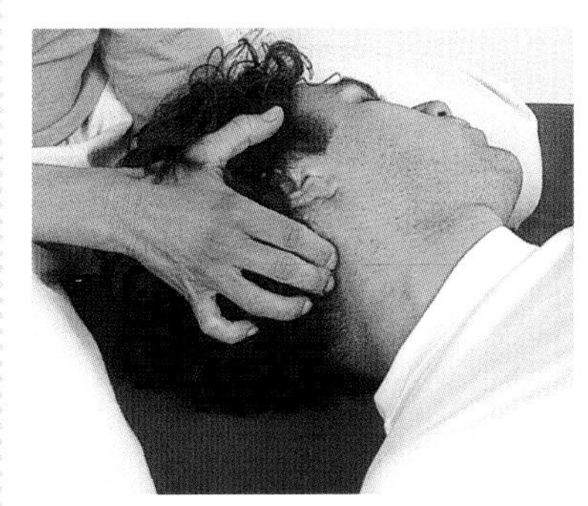

▲ Turn the head to one side and support it with one hand. Use the finger pads of your other hand to "rub" across the muscle fibres. Treat the other side of the head in the same way.

Stimulating Points Along the Base of the Skull

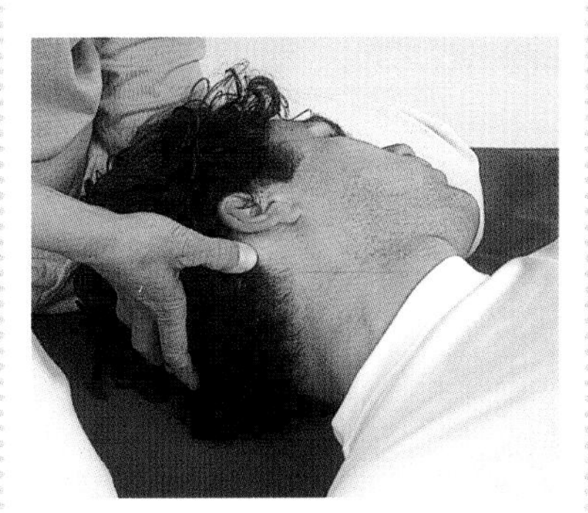

▲ With your partner's head turned to the side, press the points along the base of the skull. Start at the ear and work towards the spine. Turn the head and treat the other side in the same way.

Stimulating the Scalp

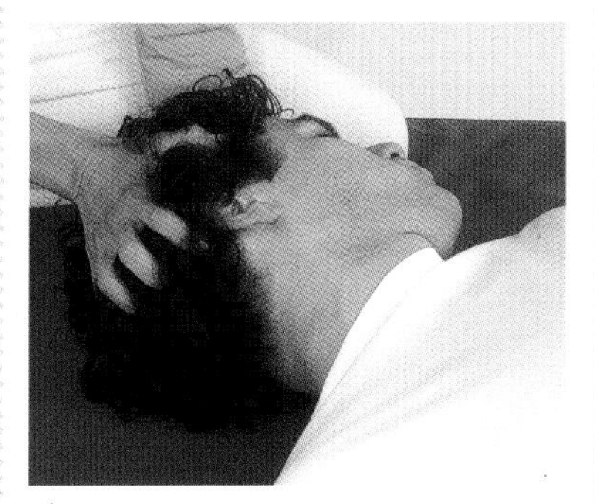

▲ Rub the scalp using your fingertips and then run your fingers through the hair.

Neck Stretch

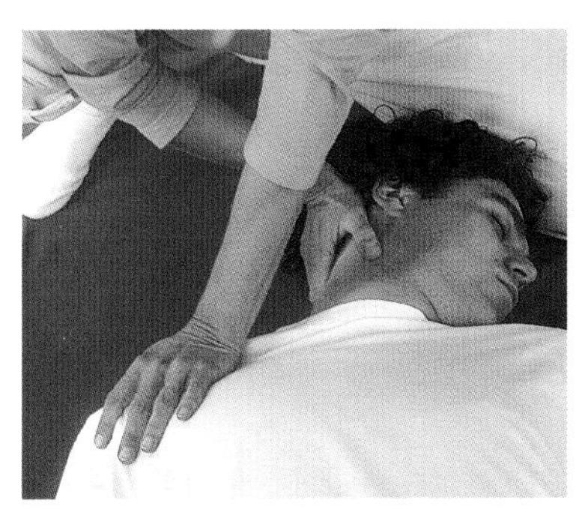

▲ Turn your partner's head to one side and support it by placing one hand at the base of the skull.

Cross your other arm over and place it on your partner's shoulder. Ask your partner to breathe in; on the out-breath, stretch this side of the neck by gently and gradually pushing the shoulder down towards the feet, keeping the other hand still. Repeat a couple of times, making sure your partner feels the stretch. Repeat on the other side of the neck.

Caution *Listen to your partner during this stretch, and take care not to cause injury.*

Treating the Face

Stroking the Forehead

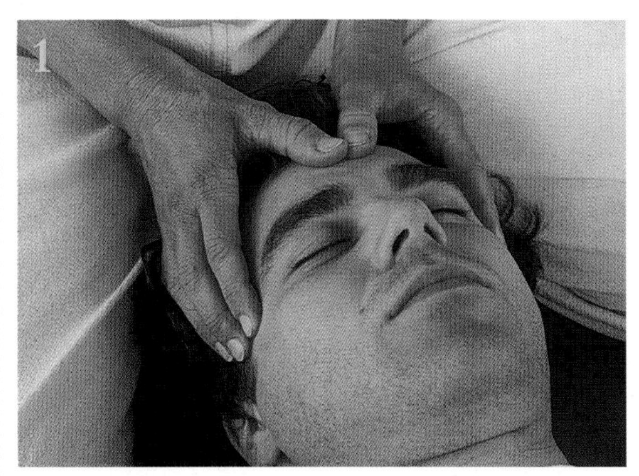

▲ Start by placing your thumbs on the midline of your partner's forehead.

▼ Apply a bit of pressure and stroke your thumbs out towards the temples. Repeat three or four times. This will ease up tension in the head and help relax the body and the mind.

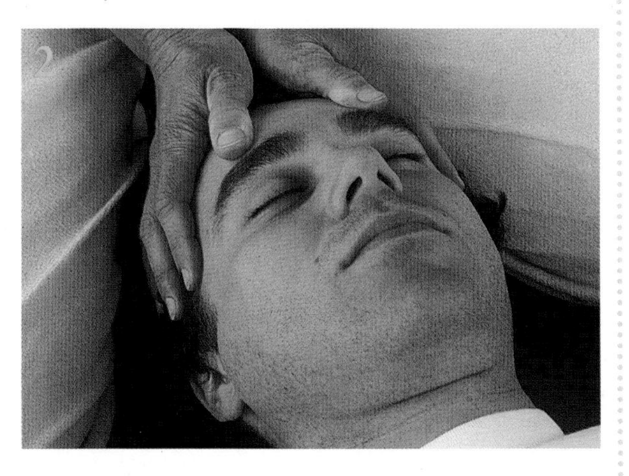

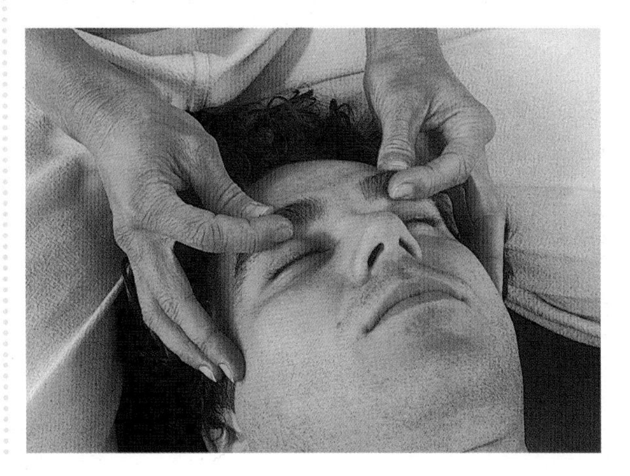

Squeezing the Eyebrows

◀ Use your index finger and thumb to squeeze your partner's eyebrows. Work from the centre out to the sides. Repeat a few times. This will help to clear sinus congestion and lift frontal headaches.

Releasing the Sinuses

▼ Using your index fingers, stroke along the side of the nose to help clear nasal congestion. Come all the way up to the bridge of the nose to stimulate point BL1, "Bright Light" with gentle pressure. BL1 is a good point to use for poor or tired vision.

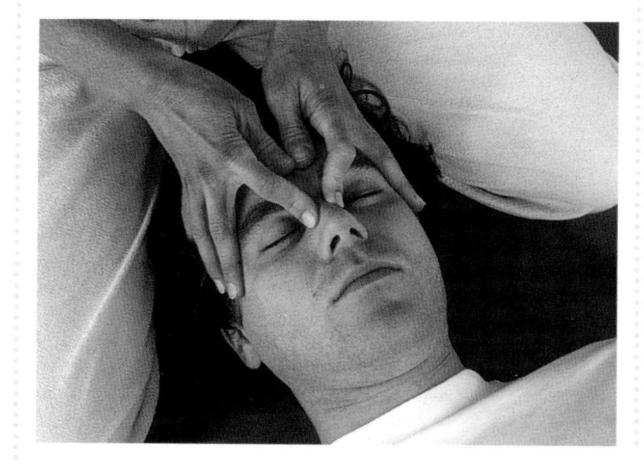

Massaging the Jaw

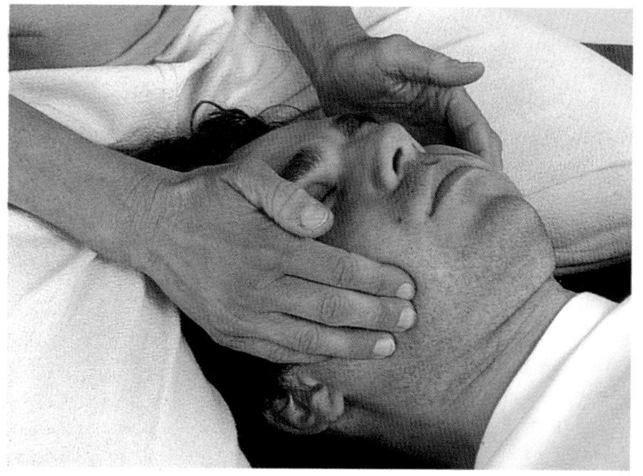

▲ Massage the side of your partner's face, moving down to the jaw. This treatment will help relax not only the face but also the whole body and will stimulate saliva production to aid digestion.

Completion

▶ Come back to the starting point at your partner's forehead. Apply some pressure using your thumbs, and gently stroke out to the sides and finish off. Give your partner time to relax after the treatment and encourage them to feel the changes in their body and mind.

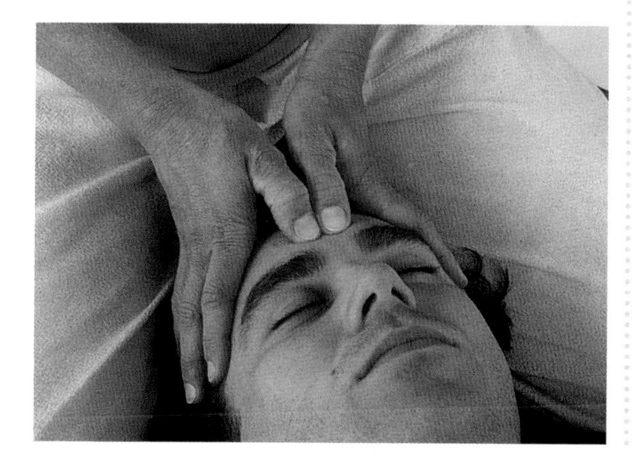

Treating Stress at your Desk

The build-up of tension and pain in the neck and shoulders are common symptoms of today's pressured and stressful work environments. The following quick-and-easy Shiatsu routine is designed for the workplace and will give relief to the accumulating tension in the neck and shoulders.

Tuning In

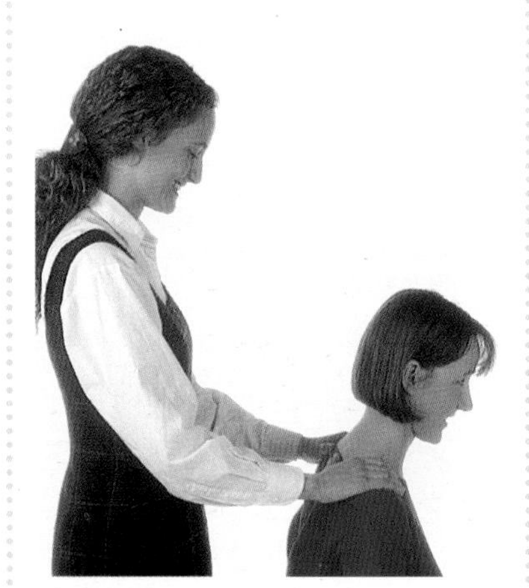

▲ Have your partner sit on a chair with proper back support to encourage a straight spine. This will allow for better energy flow. Make contact with your partner's shoulders and take a minute to tune in and see how your partner feels at this moment. Be aware of any tension your partner might hold in the shoulders and listen to the breathing.

Kneading the Shoulders

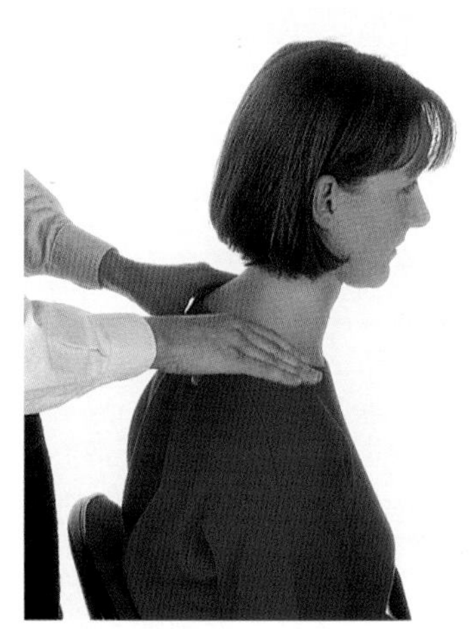

▲ Grip and hold the trapezius muscles (the muscles of the shoulders and neck) on either side of the neck. Squeeze these muscles a few times, combining your thumbs and fingers in a rhythmic "kneading" action. There may be tension initially but this will slowly dissolve. Work within your partner's pain threshold.

Lifting the Shoulders

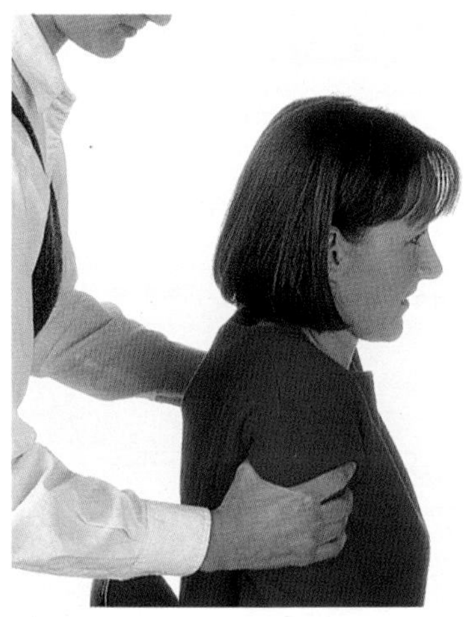

▲ To encourage your partner to relax into the treatment, take a firm grip of their upper arms; ask your partner to breathe in as you lift the shoulders up and breathe out as you allow the shoulders to drop back down again. Repeat three times.

Hacking Across the Shoulders

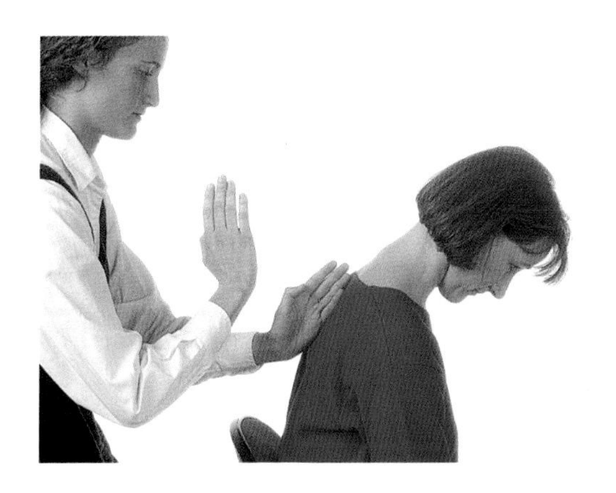

► Keep your own shoulders, wrists and hands relaxed and "soft". Use a gentle hacking action with the sides of your hands and move rhythmically across the shoulders and base of the neck. Increase the intensity and power of the hacking as the muscles relax and your partner's discomfort, if any, disappears.

1

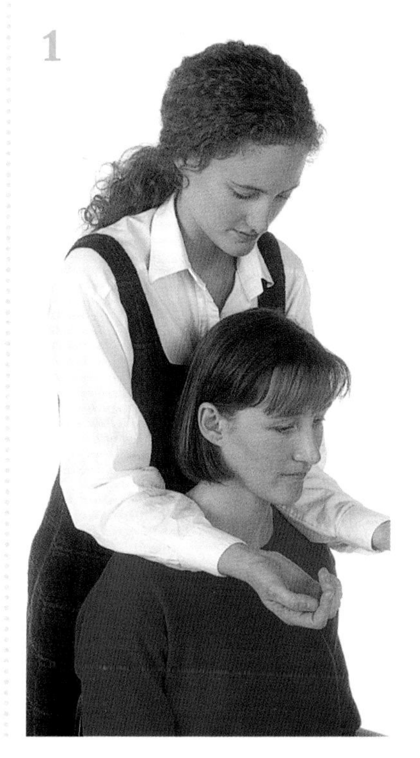

Applying Pressure to the Shoulders

◄ Stand close to your partner for support. Place your forearms on the shoulders, and on the out-breath lean into your arms, applying perpendicular pressure downwards. Repeat three times.

► Move slightly to the side. Place one hand in front and with the other thumb apply pressure to any points on top of the shoulder. Choose points you feel intuitively attracted to. These might feel sore and sensitive to start with, but as the muscle tissue gradually relaxes and the points open up, the pain will dissolve and warmth will spread across the shoulders.

2

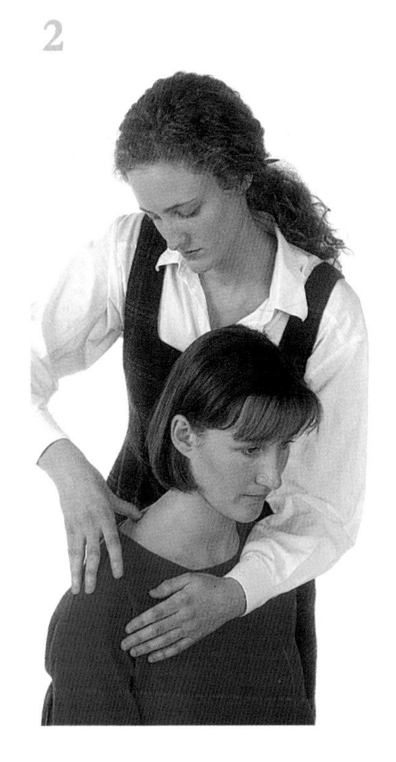

Shoulder Stretch

▶ Take hold of your partner's elbow and stretch open the shoulder by bringing the elbow across the chest. With your forearm, lean into the shoulder to increase the stretch. Shoulders are more likely to become stiff when there are problems with the digestive system. This technique will open up the energy channels running over the shoulders – Gall Bladder, Large Intestine and Small Intestine – and stimulate the digestive system into balance.

Move yourself over to the other side and treat the other shoulder in the same way.

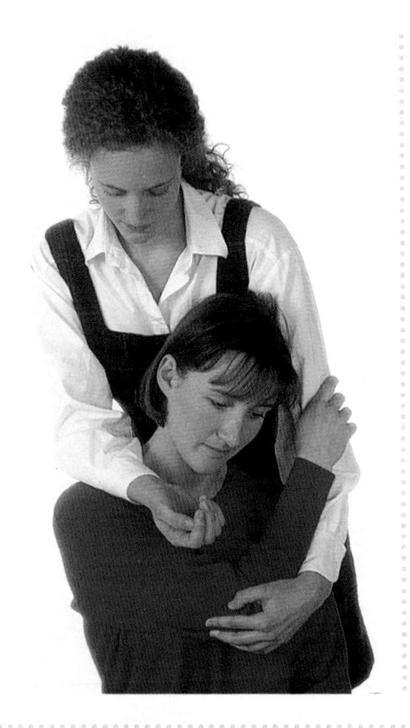

Palming the Spine

▼ Palm down your partner's spine to encourage an upright posture and stimulate the Bladder channel (affecting and calming the nervous system).

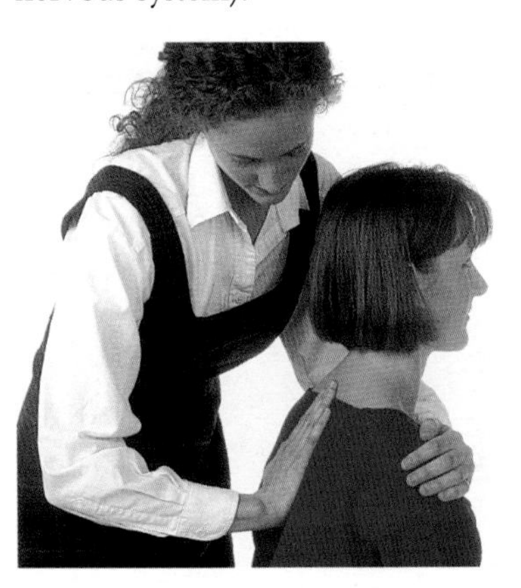

1

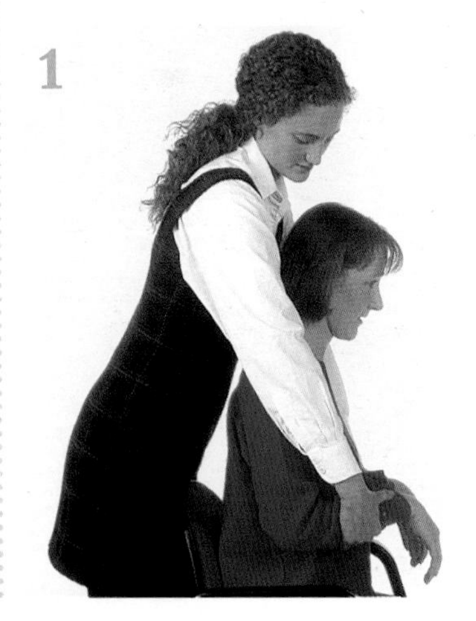

2

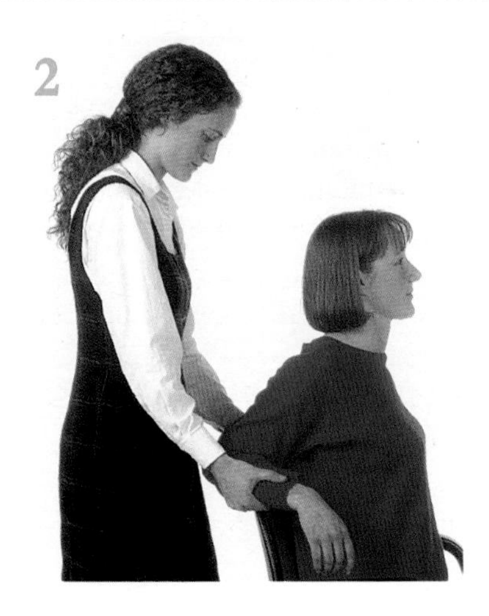

Opening of the Chest

◀ Stand behind your partner and take hold of the lower arms.

◀ Ask your partner to take a deep breath in; on the exhalation bring the elbows towards each other behind the back. Repeat three times. This will open up and expand the chest and encourage better breathing with improved posture.

Squeezing the Neck

Stand at your partner's side. Ask your partner to relax and drop the head forward into your left hand. Hold the forehead until you feel your partner has given up control of the neck. Using the fingers and thumb of your right hand, gently squeeze the muscles of the neck, patiently working from top to bottom.

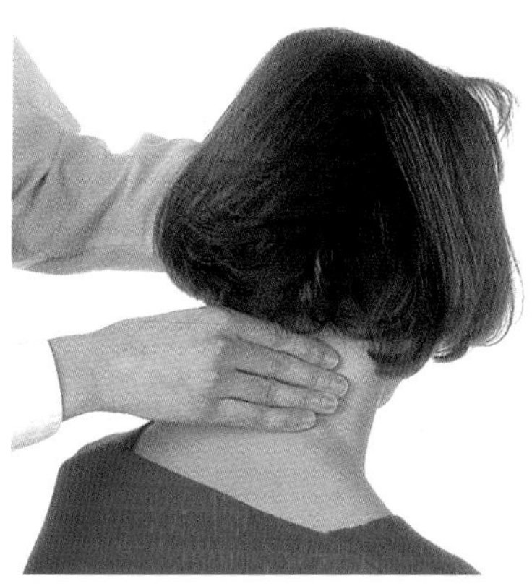

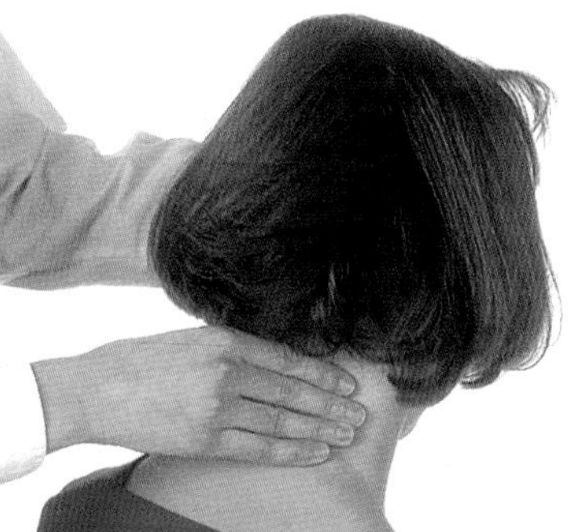

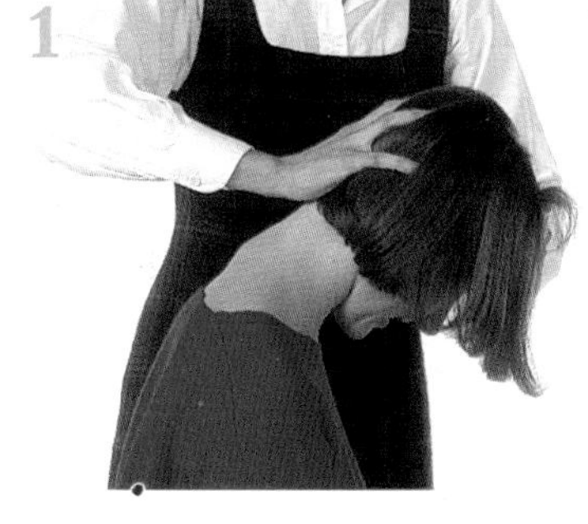

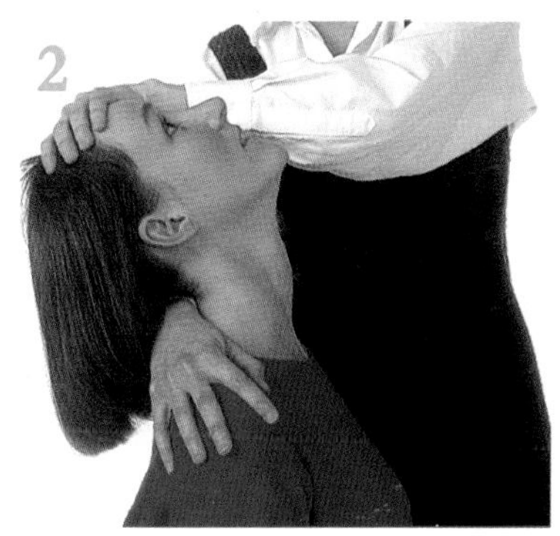

Stretching the Neck

Keep your left hand on your partner's forehead and with your right hand support the neck into a forward stretch, opening up the back of the neck and the spine.

Place your right arm across your partner's shoulders. Apply a gentle lifting movement with your forearm as your left hand guides the head backwards on to your forearm. This will stretch the front of the neck.

Caution *The base of the skull and neck must always be supported by your forearm to prevent too strong a movement backwards, which could cause injury.*

Completion

Support your partner's forehead with your left hand and bring the index finger and thumb of your right hand to the base of the skull. Imagine yourself "lifting" your partner from this position, stretching out the entire spine from sacrum to head. Ask your partner to close their eyes and hold the position for a minute, allowing your partner to feel the energy moving up and down the spine. Finish the treatment by slowly moving your hands away.

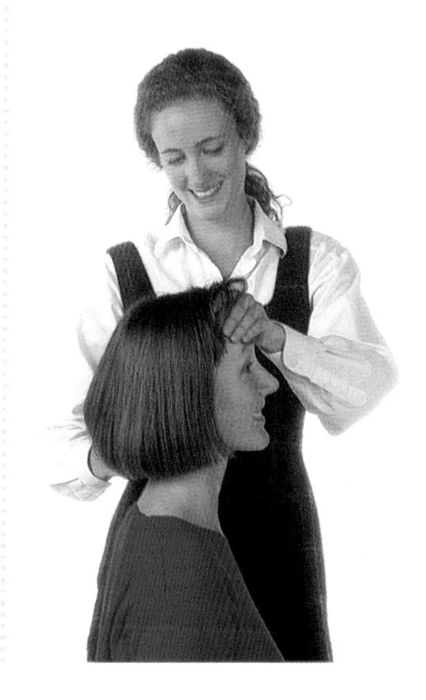

Index

Useful Addresses

To locate a Shiatsu practitioner in your local area contact: The Shiatsu Society, 31 Pulman Lane, Godalming, Surrey GU7 1XY
Tel: 01483 860771

For enquiries about studying Shiatsu in the U.K. contact: The British School of Shiatsu-Do (London), 6 Erskine Road, Primrose Hill, London NW3 3AJ. Tel: 020 7483 3776

Shiatsu Therapy Association of Australia, PO Box 598, Belgrave Vic 3160.
Tel: 03 9752 6711

New York State Society Medical Massage Therapists, Inc., PO Box 1173, Port Washington, NY 11058-0300.
Tel: 212 697 7668